Wednesday's Child

As many as one in four women have suffered severe neglect or abuse in childhood. This doubles the likelihood of their suffering clinical depression in adult life. But in spite of recent media interest in the subject, relatively little of what has been written about child-hood abuse has been based on systematic research into the lives of ordinary women.

This book summarises twenty years of research into the link between child abuse and adult depression. It breaks new ground in covering not only physical and sexual abuse but also areas which have previously received little attention, such as psychological abuse, hostile parenting and role-reversal. The reasons why such neglect and abuse occur are explored in terms of marital breakdown, poverty and parental psychiatric disorder.

The experiences of women interviewed in the course of the research are documented here in their own words. As well as demonstrating how such experience relates to adult depression among women, *Wednesday's Child* assesses the factors which can reduce the later impact of childhood abuse on both the children of today and the parents of tomorrow.

Always closely in touch with human experience, this book presents findings which have far-reaching implications not only for parents, but also for social policy-makers, social workers and other professionals involved in child protection and welfare.

Antonia Bifulco and **Patricia Moran** are both members of the social science team based at the Socio-Medical Research Centre, Royal Holloway, University of London.

Wednesday's Child

Research into women's experience
of neglect and abuse in childhood,
and adult depression

Antonia Bifulco and Patricia Moran

London and New York

First published 1998
by Routledge
11 New Fetter Lane, London EC4P 4EE

Simultaneously published in the USA and Canada
by Routledge
29 West 35th Street, New York, NY 10001

© 1998 Antonia Bifulco and Patricia Moran

Typeset in Times by J&L Composition Ltd, Filey, North Yorkshire

Printed and bound in Great Britain by MPG Books Ltd, Bodmin

British Library Cataloguing in Publication Data
A catalogue record for this book is available from the British Library

Library of Congress Cataloging in Publication Data
Bifulco, Antonia, 1955–
Wednesday's child: research into women's experience of neglect and abuse
in childhood and adult depression/Antonia Bifulco and Patricia Moran.
p. cm.
Includes bibliographical references and index.
1. Adult child abuse victims–Mental health. 2. Depression, Men-
tal.   3. Women–Mental health.
I. Moran, Patricia, 1960–
II. Title.
RC569.5.C55B54   1998
616.85'27071'082–dc21

                                                                97–26564
                                                                CIP

ISBN 0–415–16526–1 (hbk)
ISBN 0–415–16527–X (pbk)

This book is dedicated to our husbands, Vincent and Peter, for providing encouragement, support and a secure base. It is also dedicated to our daughters, Lucy and Eleanor, neither of whom were born on a Wednesday. We hope they will benefit from what we have learned!

Contents

Preface

Myths, folklore and superstitions bear eloquent testimony to man's age-old intuition that events occurring in infancy and childhood, or even prenatally, may determine the subsequent course of life . . . Thousands of years were to elapse before that intuition was to be scientifically approached.

(Furst 1967: 3)[1]

The purpose of this book is to make available to a wider readership the accounts of childhood trauma we have collected in the course of researching the links between early experience and clinical depression in adult life. For many it may seem intuitive, and thus unnecessary to prove scientifically, that early experiences influence what happens to us as adults. But the world of the child and adolescent is complex, encompassing a variety of potentially influential experiences in the first sixteen years of life. Harmful experiences do not necessarily come singly, neither do they exist in a vacuum devoid of any happier ones. Intuitive understanding cannot hope to grasp the complex mechanisms by which various interrelated childhood experiences influence different adult outcomes. Systematic research is required to disentangle the elements of adverse experience responsible for the greatest impact. Such investigation is also required to clarify the differences between one form of abuse and another, and to assess the severity of abuse required for an experience to have lasting rather than short-term impact. More optimistically, systematic study can hope eventually to pinpoint which particular positive experiences give most protection against long-term negative consequences.

The study of childhood neglect and abuse in relation to adult disorder often requires highly technical analyses in which the individual case histories and descriptions of the phenomena are overlooked. The experiences described in the following chapters seek to both illustrate and summarise the results of research conducted by one particular research team over the last two decades. For those wishing to pursue the scientific evidence, full references to more technical publications together with details of findings and samples are provided in the notes to each chapter and the Appendices. Our aim here is to illustrate the findings of our team rather than to attempt to give coverage of the vast array of research by other workers in this area.

Our research involved face-to-face interviews with women recalling their life histories. These interviews proved to have a double benefit in advancing knowledge. First, systematic, statistical study made on the basis of the material has led to scientific publications available to practitioners in the fields of social science and psychiatry. Second, the interviews themselves provide an oral history of the lives of over 800 women, reflecting a historical period of half a century stretching back to the end of the First World War. The summary of these findings, illustrated with rich case history accounts, are presented here in a form we hope is readily accessible to both lay and professional readers. These descriptions of the key experiences that have moulded women's lives have lain dormant for many years in university filing cabinets. We wanted to revive these abandoned accounts and let the descriptions tell the story of how childhood and adult experience are linked.

The accounts are based on research projects conducted since the late 1970s by the research team at Royal Holloway (formerly Bedford College), University of London directed by George Brown. All the projects focused on the experience of London women, all of whom were ordinary members of the public. While over a third of the women were selected for having had adverse childhood or adult experience, most of the remainder were representative of people in urban British settings. The interviews were usually conducted in the women's own homes, surroundings in which they were comfortable and could talk openly about their experiences. The childhood material was questioned about by means of the 'Childhood Experience of Care and Abuse' (CECA) instrument, a semi-structured interview which allows women to talk freely about their childhood experience in chronological sequence from earliest years.[2] Even though some of their experiences were distressing to recount, the women often expressed relief that their accounts were believed, and seemed pleased to have the chance to speak to an outsider in confidence about what they viewed as important life experiences. They were highly committed to the research and gave many hours of their time to be interviewed. They understood the importance of tracing links between childhood and adult experience and appreciated that other women might be helped by it in the future. We hope that this book will reflect the generosity of these women, and will have a beneficial influence on those who, unlike researchers, have to remedy the ill-effects of child abuse such as policy-makers, social workers, teachers and medical staff.

. The emphasis of this book is on childhood neglect and abuse, so many of the stories recounted are sad and painful. However, not all the childhood experiences were unhappy and the reader should bear in mind that we have selected the more severe ones linked with adult disorder in order to illustrate associations found in the analyses. The stories were not uniformly bleak. Accounts of childhood varied in terms of the balance of negative and positive experiences, and although we have focused more on the former here, we have also tried to assess the positive influences. We found instances of care, concern and companionship from parents, as well as support from other adults in childhood promoting enjoyment and fun. In adulthood we found instances of strength, courage, resilience, humour and perseverance, paradoxically often alongside vulnerability. This is the reason why women who suffered childhood abuse are often termed 'survivors'. Investigating the long-term ill-effects of such early experience goes hand in hand with investigating resilience or 'damage limitation' in terms of adult functioning. People often ask whether it is depressing to hear these accounts. Surprisingly, this is rarely the case. What typically remains after contact with the interviewed women is less the sadness of the story and more the impression of resilience in coping with adversity. These women all survived to tell their stories and voiced their determination to improve circumstances for their own children and future generations.

The 'Wednesday's child (is full of woe)' appellation is, of course, based on the well-known nursery rhyme which declares that the day of the week on which a child is born determines its future fate. Certainly for most of the women we saw there seemed a chance element to the damaging circumstances into which they were born and over which they had little control during childhood years. However in later years many went on to 'earn' security in the form of supportive relationships, successful careers, a sense of mastery over their adult lives and a fierce commitment to their own children, helped by those close to them. A somewhat less well-known children's rhyme gives a different account of the influence of days of the week: 'Monday for wealth, Tuesday for health and Wednesday the best day of all'. Many of the accounts we heard showed a similar switch – often as a result of supportive relationships – from woeful beginnings to later well-being.

NOTES

1 Furst, S. (1967) *Psychic Trauma*, London: Basic Books.
2 Bifulco, A., Brown, G.W. and Harris, T. (1995) 'Childhood experience of care and abuse: a retrospective interview measure', *Journal of Child Psychology and Psychiatry 35*: 1419–1435.

Acknowledgements

The studies reported in this book represent twenty years of research undertaken by a social science team based at the Socio-Medical Research Centre in Bedford Square, Royal Holloway (formerly Bedford College), University of London. This work has been carried out under the directorship of Professor George Brown, OBE, whose distinctive approach to social research on depression has been successfully funded for over two decades, together with Tirril Harris who was responsible for first placing childhood experience on the research team's agenda. The research itself would not have been possible without a team of dedicated researchers who worked hard to collect the data on the several projects, in particular to Sue Adler and Bernice Andrews for developing parts of the 'Childhood Experience of Care and Abuse' (CECA) instrument, Laurence Letchford for his computing skills and Tom Craig for advice on psychiatric ratings.

We are grateful to the Medical Research Council for their generous support over the years. We also thank the John D. and Catherine T. MacArthur Foundation (Network for Development and Psychopathology) for additional financial help in developing the CECA instrument and training package, through the enthusiastic support of Dr David Kupfer and Dr Ellen Frank of Pittsburgh, USA. We would like to thank Helen Thomas and Maggie Moran for their help and advice in getting this book published and to Caroline Ball for her helpful comments on the manuscript. We are particularly indebted to Odette Bernazzani for her encouragement and support and her very valuable contribution to the presentation of material and ideas in this book. We would also like to thank Pauline Moran for her patient, affectionate care of Eleanor during the writing of the manuscript.

We are grateful to several general practitioners in Islington and Walthamstow for access to their lists of patients. Naturally none of this work would have been possible without the generous help of the women themselves who were interviewed. As always we are in their debt.

Monday's child is fair of face,
Tuesday's child is full of grace,
Wednesday's child is full of woe,
Thursday's child has far to go,
Friday's child is loving and giving,
Saturday's child works hard for a living;
And the child that is born on the Sabbath day,
Is fair and wise and good and gay.

Chapter 1

Introduction: history-taking

> The patient comes with a story, however tentative and disjointed, which is then worked on by therapist and patient until a more coherent and satisfying narrative emerges which provides an objectification and explanation of the patient's difficulties, and a vehicle . . . which links inner and outer experiences.
>
> (Holmes 1993: 158)[1]

Most people are of the opinion that experiences in childhood have a lasting impact. Indeed, many adults can identify particular experiences occurring in their formative years which they believe have helped to shape the person they have become. Knowing precisely *which* experiences are influential and how they have effect is a matter for systematic investigation by social scientists and others. Our research team has been exploring the effects of early experience for two decades, with particular interest in its relationship to clinical depression in adulthood. By interviewing women about their childhood it has been possible to identify a range of experiences which increase the chances of depression occurring in adult life. As expected, the types of experiences that play a significant role in this process are those involving neglect and abuse.

For the majority of children the quality of care that parents provide, if not perfect, is adequate for their mental and physical well-being. Nevertheless, it is clear that parental care is seriously deficient for a significant number of children, as evidenced by the large numbers of children placed on child protection registers annually. Figures for England show that as many as 28,000 children were *added* to the register in 1996.[2] These are children known to be subjected to sexual, physical or emotional abuse or neglect. The scale of the problem is likely to be larger when we take into account the numbers of neglected and abused children that never get reported, the children who suffer in silence. Most of us are horrified at the thought of such abuse, and as a society we are probably more concerned and have more agencies attempting to alleviate such suffering of children than at any time in history.

Being on the receiving end of neglect and abuse is obviously distressing and painful for the child at the time it occurs. In addition the long-term damage caused by such experiences can be equally dire, thwarting psychological and social development. Under some conditions this results in individuals entering adulthood too damaged to cope with the demands of everyday living and raising the next generation of children. But do most of us know exactly what constitutes neglect and abuse? Would most of us be able to differentiate parental behaviour that is perhaps impatient, insensitive or overly lax from that which is abusive? Do we know the conditions under which abuse occurs or the extent of the associated psychological damage in adulthood? Despite much debate there is a need for research to establish the precise nature of the relationship between childhood maltreatment and adult outcomes. It is required to inform not only professionals working in the childcare field but also parents and teachers responsible for their own and other children's welfare. It may also be useful for individuals seeking to understand their own lives in terms of their early experiences.

This book sets out to enhance understanding of child neglect and abuse, and to investigate its long-term effects with particular emphasis on adult depression, one of the most common emotional disorders in women. It draws upon our research findings to present a summary of the key experiences occurring in childhood which are capable of making an impact in adulthood. We examine the circumstances associated with such challenging experiences in order to begin to unravel some of the causes of child abuse. In this vein we explore how parents under stress, who may be coping with troubled marriages, reconstituted families, poverty and their own psychiatric disorder, may influence a child's upbringing. While the outcome of main interest involves adult depression, along the route we examine other factors associated with abusive childhood experience such as low self-esteem and a lack of supportive relationships.

THE STUDY OF LIFE-TIME EXPERIENCE

The approach we adopted in studying the influence of childhood was a biographical one, based on 'history-taking' interviews with adult women. It was Winnicott who described psychotherapy as an 'extended form of history-taking'.[3] While our aim was not one of providing psychotherapy, our approach was similar insofar as we were interested in collecting detailed information laden with both context and meaning for the individual. As in the process described in the title quote, we too aimed to examine such stories to see how the adverse early environment inflicted damage on the child's and then the adult's inner and outer world.

We documented the experiences arising throughout the life course which might create either risk for, or protection against, a woman's chance of developing depression. We adopted this approach not only because we felt it constituted the most thorough measurement of these experiences but also because it aided theoretical understanding. Thus we hoped that by encouraging women to tell their life histories in their own words and by using their quotes in this book, we could generate empathic understanding of the experience of early neglect and abuse and the damage that it inflicts. We also felt we had much to learn from the interviewed women. In this we followed John Bowlby who wrote: 'Whilst some traditional therapists might be described as advocating the stance "I know: I'll tell you", the stance I advocate is one of "You know, you tell me."'[4]

Prior work by our research team had shown that episodes of depression are fairly common, with one in ten working-class mothers developing a new episode of depression in any one year. These episodes are associated with crises occurring in their lives typically involving losses, humiliations, rejections or increasing entrapment in punishing situations. Typical crises involve a husband leaving for another woman, a teenage son in trouble with the police, or the family in an overcrowded flat being refused rehousing. In inner-London boroughs where much of the research took place, such crises are common, affecting over a third of women in any one year.[5] Following such crises a fifth of women are likely to become depressed. This means, of course, that the majority do *not* experience clinical depression in response to such crises. We sought to investigate the reasons why one in five were particularly susceptible to depression and the remaining four protected. On further investigation it was discovered that, prior to becoming depressed, a number of features made women vulnerable to the unpleasant effects of a crisis. These included low self-esteem, a discordant relationship with partner or children, and lack of support from friends or relatives.

Conversely, women with higher self-esteem and good support survived similar crises without becoming seriously depressed.[6]

We set about tracing the origins of such adult vulnerability, and began our search in childhood. We wanted to know, for example, if a woman who finds herself in a relationship with an unresponsive partner, or who finds herself unable to relate to her children is more likely to have been mistreated by her parents when she was a child. We did not, however, expect *all* adult vulnerability to stem from childhood; we saw that almost anyone could experience difficulties in relationships in adult life which made them temporarily susceptible to depressive disorder. However, we expected that women with more enduring vulnerability emanating from childhood would show signs of greater psychological scarring and disadvantage. They would have a somewhat different experience of depression: their episodes would be more severe and last longer, and they would have repeated depressions throughout their life, with the earliest starting in teenage years.

We also wanted to examine the other side of the coin: that for some an adverse childhood may lead to a strength and resilience perhaps not found in those with uneventful or over-protected early years. The expression 'earned security' describes how such women learn to overcome their early life disadvantages. We needed simultaneously to investigate factors which were damaging and those which were protective against the effects of mistreatment. Thus themes of both susceptibility and strengthening required exploration.

GENDER

Our decision to study women rather than men was in the first instance a pragmatic one: rates of clinical depression among women are nearly double that of men.[7] This is not to say that the experiences of boys and fathers should not be similarly documented. Research has shown that men similarly suffer neglect and abuse and these also link with adult psychiatric disorders. However, there are differences which require a more detailed investigation than is possible here. These include important differences in the type of childhood experiences, as well as differences in response to maltreatment. Thus adolescent boys have higher rates of delinquent behaviour and alcohol or drug abuse than girls, and have a much higher rate of suicide in young adulthood. Exploring gender differences is complex, and we wanted to avoid introducing this additional element in developing a preliminary model of childhood experience and adult psychiatric disorder. Hence this book is devoted to female experience.

THE STUDY OF CHILDHOOD

We began our work on childhood experience with no fully developed theory in mind. This allowed us to throw our net wide, and measure as full a context of relevant experience as possible. In the early stages of our work we were influenced by the writings of two eminent workers in the field: John Bowlby and Michael Rutter. From John Bowlby we adopted the notion that loss of mother in childhood and disrupted family relationships interfere with a child's later ability to form close, loving relationships.[8] From Michael Rutter we learned that a conflictful and stressful environment in a child's early years leads to a perpetuation of adverse circumstances into adult life.[9, 10] The first emphasised the internal damage suffered by the child, the second the effects of a wider hostile environment. To make sense of the relationship between childhood experience and adult depression, we attempted to bring these two ideas together. This approach took into account not only negative psychological states such as low self-esteem, helplessness and poor ability to relate to others but also the interaction of these with the very real adversities present in the external world. These included economic hardship, the breakdown of family life and disadvantages associated with lower social class position. We felt it was essential to look at the interface between such deprived inner and outer worlds to understand vulnerability to depression.

We chose to interview adult women about their memories of childhood experience rather than attempt to question children directly. We had a number of reasons for this. First, we could collect all the information about a woman's life history without waiting years to assess what happened to her as she grew up. Second, we felt that the accounts we obtained retrospectively were more comprehensive than those we could have obtain by interviewing children at the time of their abuse. Consider, for example, how difficult it would be for an eight-year-old girl to describe ongoing sexual abuse to an interviewer. Would she understand the questions? Would threats from the abuser have placed her in fear of her life if she told us about the abuse? Interviewing children about their experiences is full of such pitfalls. We felt we were more likely to obtain an accurate description of these experiences by interviewing adult women, when they were old enough to understand the experience and could recount the abuse without fear. We also knew that interviewing children who might have been recently abused would have raised major ethical considerations. Not only would it put the child under unbearable pressure in terms of whether to disclose the information, but it would have changed our research activity into an intervention programme – a worthy aim, but one which we were not qualified or funded to undertake.

MEMORY OF CHILDHOOD

We thus adopted a historical retrospective approach, measuring reports of experiences that happened years ago. We were among the first in the late 1970s to tackle such a long recall period and it was viewed at first with some scepticism by parts of the scientific community. It was argued that people had poor memory of child-hood experience, and that recollections would be distorted. Such distortion would arise because people's memories would be coloured by their *feelings* towards parents and other family members which would render the collection of accurate, fac-tual information on childhood virtually impossible. It was also claimed that distortion of childhood memories would arise due to symptoms of depression. It was expected that, on the one hand, depressed women would give an account of childhood biased towards a particularly negative view of their experience, and on the other hand, non-depressed women would give an account of childhood that was biased towards a particularly 'rosy' view. The exercise, it was argued, would be futile.

We attempted to overcome this problem through very careful and detailed measurement. In our history-taking interviews we concen-trated on the *factual* aspects of women's childhood experience. We wanted to know as precisely as possible what had occurred, how often, at what age and with whom. This involved going beyond the more subjective feelings women had about the way they were treated in childhood, and probing for 'hard evidence' in the form of detailed examples. Although we were interested in the impact of such experience in childhood, we had to show that the women's feelings were rooted in actual and not imagined experiences. For example, if a woman said she *felt* her mother wasn't interested in her upbringing we explored the statement further rather than accepting it at face value. We probed for details both of the care she received in terms of whether she had regular meals and clean clothes, who prepared them, how often, and so on, as well as questioning about her mother's critical and rejecting behaviour. In this way we built up a body of information illustrated with actual instances of behaviour which was distinct from the women's subjective feelings about what had occurred. This enabled us to compare childhoods, to see if those women who had the *most* adverse childhoods were also the most likely to experience depression in adulthood.

From the outset we believed it was possible that women could recall significant events in childhood and be keen to recount them. It would at the very least give the women a chance for their experiences to be listened to and believed. We made certain assumptions about people's ability to recall their childhood memories. First, we assumed that the more significant experiences in childhood were less likely to have been forgotten than the more routine or trivial happenings. For example, we thought that most people would know the age they were when their mother died or their father left home, but may not recall each birthday party or school exam. Second, we believed that the recall of early memories would be enhanced if asked about in chronological sequence with earlier memories triggering later ones. Certain anchoring dates were used to help map out experiences, such as starting primary or secondary school or births of siblings. Third, we considered that if a woman had enough time to give considered answers, it would be possible to reconstruct in the interview a faithful account of what occurred in her childhood. Hence interviews sometimes lasted several hours and it was not uncommon for women to recall incidents that they had not attended to for years. At times women also revised their view of the sequence of experiences when they reconstructed all their memories for that period of time. For example one woman thought she had been separated from her mother before she started school, then suddenly had a memory of being taken to school by her mother, and realised that it had all occurred a year or two later than she had previously believed.

We had to consider that for certain topics it was possible that not all of these principles of remembering would apply. For example, sexual abuse, although a significant experience, may be hampered in its recall by the sexual ignorance of the child at the time. The experience may never have been coded in memory as sexual abuse. In some instances, women sexually abused at a very young age recreated its meaning subsequently. Sometimes the painful nature of an experience might have pushed the memory out of a woman's conscious mind for so long that recounting the incident was difficult. Although many struggled to find the right words, and their stories were at times disjointed, most women were able to give full accounts of childhood experience including sexual abuse.

In recent years the debate concerning fabricated memories or 'false memory syndrome' has received much attention. Allegations that psychotherapists use suggestion to assist their patients in 'remembering' sexual abuse which never actually took place have been tested with litigation in the United States.[11] This echoes Freud's claims earlier this century that his patients' childhood sexual abuse were fantasies, a position heavily criticised by a later generation.[12] The pendulum of public opinion concerning the truth or not of childhood abuse continues to swing back and forth. In terms of our research interviews, we had no reason to disbelieve the women's accounts of their experiences. After all, they had no prior knowledge of the research ideas we were testing and had no motive for giving us anything other than the truth. Many were simply glad to have the opportunity to disclose information about their early adverse experience. Only a minority had been in psychotherapy, and when we first started the research, few would have encountered discussions of abuse in the media. However, we nevertheless looked for corroborating evidence and in order to gain a second version of childhood from the same family, we intentionally interviewed a large number of pairs of sisters. Each sister was interviewed separately and confidentially by different interviewers who recorded the information without reference to the other interview. The high degree of similarity of the sisters' accounts of their own and each other's childhood experiences reported in this book confirms that the women's accounts were likely to be accurate.

A more common obstacle in gathering childhood histories was not fabrication, or exaggeration of accounts, but rather the reverse. Often women wanted to 'normalise' or minimise the severity of their negative experiences. They wished to portray their parents and others in a more positive light than any outsider would have done. Many strove to excuse parents or carers for their neglectful and abusive behaviours. We found that under-reporting of abuse rather than fabrication was potentially more of a problem. Because of this possibility we questioned about any abuse, however minor, in case these proved to be of significance in the analysis. We never discounted, for example, a report of hitting in the family simply because the woman claimed it to be 'normal' for that place and time. We recorded all potential instances of abuse in the same way regardless of the woman's interpretations or justifications.

OUR RESEARCH PROJECTS

We decided to investigate the experiences of women living in the community rather than depressed patients in hospital settings, where much research on depression is conducted. There were a number of reasons for this choice. First, we thought it likely that experiences of neglect and abuse were more common in the community at large than was generally believed. Our analyses would provide an estimate of how common these experiences were. Second, we needed women *without* either abusive childhoods or depression for comparison purposes. Third, we were also interested in women who in spite of experiencing adverse childhoods did *not* become depressed. This group of women might provide insights into experiences that protect women from depression. Fourth, we knew that there was a good deal of psychiatric disorder, particularly depression, which was never treated by psychiatrists or even general practitioners. These women would have been 'missing' from our research had we focused solely on those who sought treatment.

The childhood case histories referred to in subsequent chapters are taken from four separate research projects, conducted between 1977 and 1995, each project lasting between three and five years. (Full details of samples are given in Appendix I.) Overall, just over 800 women were interviewed about their childhood and adult lives. The aims of the projects varied, but a major component of each project was to investigate the relationship between childhood experience and adult depression. Two projects involved women selected by questionnaire for the presence of adversity in childhood. The first project, the 'Loss of Mother Study', began in 1977 and investigated the consequences of losing a parent in childhood. In 1990 the 'Sisters Study' selected 100 women for interview, over half of whom had been neglected or abused in childhood, and each of whom had a sister who was also interviewed to give another separate account of the family's history. In 1990 a third study, the 'Adult Risk' project, selected women because they had negative *adult* experiences related to depression. This project studied just over 100 women who were vulnerable to depression through ongoing poor self-esteem, conflictful family relationships, and lack of supportive relationships outside the home. This provided an opportunity to see how these factors may have derived from adversity in childhood. For comparison purposes nearly 300 women in the 1980 'Representative London Women' sample, all of whom were either working-class mothers or single parents, were selected regardless of childhood or adult risk experience. This provided figures for the prevalence of adverse childhood experiences in a relatively typical, inner-city population of mothers. Across the four projects we had collected a wide variety of childhood histories ranging from those who had experienced gross neglect and abuse, to those who had very positive experiences with their parents.

DEFINING CHILDHOOD TRAUMA

One of the major problems of research into childhood experience concerns the precise definition of abuse. The way in which experiences are identified as either harmful or harmless, disadvantageous or positively beneficial, was often a question of degree. For example, if we consider disciplinary practices, imposing discipline by means of serious beatings and physical injury is easily identified as damaging, whereas other less harsh and more flexible means of enforcing discipline, such as imposing sanctions against the child, are commonly believed to be not only harmless but positively beneficial. However, at the other extreme, the effects of lax discipline are harder to predict. The boundaries between these experiences needed to be defined in our own research. It was also unclear at the outset how severe a childhood experience had to be in order to cause psychological or other damage in years to come. Many parents, at times of high irritation, give their child a single slap or make critical or hurtful remarks. Others may beat their child relentlessly until injuries are sustained, or tell their child on a daily basis how much it is unloved and unwanted. Whereas most would judge the former as constituting normal, if undesirable, parent–child relations, most would also agree on the likely adverse effects of the latter. However, there remains a grey area between these extremes about which little is known. Through our research we hoped to be able to show precisely how much hitting or criticism had to take place before long-term damage was incurred.

The experiences we had in mind as constituting abuse typically involved failure to meet the child's needs for safety, belonging and being valued. Thus neglect and physical attack jeopardised safety, while humiliation and exploitation of the child undermined a sense of belonging and value. The more childhood histories we collected, the better we were able to categorise each experience. We began by examining the impact of losing a parent, and explored the consequences for the child in terms of neglect by replacement parents, and of exploitation through the related experience of role-reversal. We learnt from this that antipathy, rejection and physical abuse were common in neglectful households. We progressed to exploring sexual abuse, and only came more latterly to conceptualise psychological abuse as a further category of exploitative and domineering parenting.

SELF-ESTEEM, COPING AND RELATIONS WITH OTHERS

One of the key aims of the research was to explore the links between childhood adversity, poor self-esteem, poor coping and the failure to develop close relationships with others. These latter factors are known to relate to depression and we were interested in whether their origins could be traced back to the early years of life. We therefore questioned about damage to self-esteem in childhood in terms of feelings of inferiority, and about poor coping in terms of helplessness. We also asked about how experiences impacted on perceptions of self in relation to others in terms of childhood feelings of shame, loneliness and social isolation. Since our research focused on social and psychological factors, we were unable to explore the possible role of genetic, physiological, temperamental and constitutional factors in explaining these differences. While there is little doubt that these play a role in increasing risk for depression, our contribution lies in enhancing understanding of the psychological factors interfacing between the individual and a hostile social world.

DEPRESSION IN ADULTHOOD

For the sake of simplicity the outcome that we have focused on here is adult depression occurring in a twelve-month period before interview. In two of the four projects a prospective or forward-looking design was used with women interviewed on more than one occasion, so that factors preceding the onset of depression in the year could be explored. We did not assess depression of the bipolar variety ('manic depression'), nor the endogenous type more commonly found in hospital settings. We were interested in the more common neurotic disorder. Where we collected additional information about episodes of depression occurring across the lifespan from teenage years onwards, we found largely similar results to those reported for the twelve-month period. In order to assess whether the women we interviewed had been depressed in the prior year, we used a well-known psychiatric assessment.[13] We were interested in the depression at a severe or 'clinical' level which would be disabling in terms of normal activities. This was distinct from the more common lower grade depressions experienced by most people from time to time. Although the latter might similarly involve feeling low and sad, they have less intensity and fewer accompanying symptoms than a full clinical disorder. Severely depressed people typically hold a triad of negative views whereby the self is seen as worthless, the world as meaningless and the future as pointless.[14] This level of depression cannot be easily shaken off, and is likely to interfere with everyday functioning.

To convey the severity of the depressive disorders we encountered, the following is an example of depression experienced by one woman: 'I hated myself, I hated my job, I hated the people I worked with. I just felt like I hated everything and everyone around me. I didn't know if I was coming or going. I really thought I was having a nervous breakdown. I would cry every night. I had no one to talk to. I couldn't eat, I lost two and a half stone in weight and didn't sleep more that a couple of hours a night. I would walk up and down in my bedroom, or read a book until four o'clock in the morning.' She was unable to concentrate at work, lost interest in everything including her appearance, and felt tired and slowed down in her movements. She felt hopeless about the future and made a suicide attempt: 'I don't know how I managed to get through that time. I nearly didn't. I took an overdose of paracetamol. I felt I couldn't take any more, that I was on my own, that I couldn't talk to anyone.' The episode lasted around nine months and she never approached a doctor for treatment.

CONTENT OF CHAPTERS

This book is divided into three parts: the first explores experiences of neglect involving parental indifference, role-reversal and antipathy to the child. The second part concerns varieties of abuse: physical, sexual and psychological. Although these mainly involve parental behaviour they also cover a wider range of perpetrators including other household members and those outside the household. The third and final part explores the family context of neglect and abuse and its long-term outcomes in both teenage years and adult life, as well as positive factors which reduce vulnerability and depression.

Four points should be made clear which apply to all the childhood experiences discussed in this book. The first is that by 'childhood' we mean all the early years of life up to the end of the sixteenth year, thus including early teenage years. Second, the experiences we cover occurred in various family arrangements, not only with natural parents. Thus the term 'parent' refers to the primary caregivers in the home whether natural or replacement parent figures. Each chapter examines whether particular negative experiences were more common in different types of family structure. Third, loss of parent prior to such family arrangements was defined in terms of either death of parent or separation from parent for twelve months or more for any reason, not only parental divorce. Fourth, within each chapter examples are given of maltreatment graded as 'marked', 'moderate' or 'mild' in order to show the full range of experience reported. However, since it emerged that 'mild' instances of neglect or abuse did not relate to significant levels of long-term damage, for most of the analyses (including prevalence rates) only those judged to be 'marked' or 'moderate' are referred to. Those with mild abuse are combined with those who had no neglect or abuse.

The first two sections of this book cover six different, but related, adverse childhood experiences each selected because of an association with adult depression. Each can be seen incontrovertibly as an adult infringement of children's rights. The effects of adults ignoring children's needs for material and emotional care were examined in terms of neglect and role reversal. The use of oppressive rather than reasonable control was examined in terms of antipathy, physical and psychological abuse. Misuse of power over children was investigated in terms of sexual abuse. The effects of these on self-esteem, coping and relationships with others in childhood, and the association between childhood neglect or abuse and depression in adulthood are discussed in each chapter. Each of the chapters also examines the degree of corroboration provided by a hundred pairs of sisters raised together but interviewed independently, to check on the accuracy of information.

This also allowed for an estimate of how often such experiences were shared by siblings.

The third section broadens the discussion to consider the inter-relationship of different forms of neglect or abuse and the family contexts in which these experiences most often occur. We also trace the effects of childhood adversity throughout the life course: its impact on teenage and adult vulnerability in terms of adult low self-esteem, poor coping and poor support are examined. Finally the likely protective effects of experiences at different points in the life course are discussed. The implications of this research in terms of social policy, parenting and education are then explored in the conclusion.

NOTES

1 Holmes, J. (1993) *John Bowlby and Attachment Theory*, London: Routledge.
2 NSPCC (1996) *Children and Young People on Child Protection Registers in England*, London: Government Statistical Office.
3 Winnicott, D. (1965) *The Maturational Process and the Facilitating Environment*, London: Hogarth.
4 Bowlby, J. (1988) *A Secure Base: Clinical Applications of Attachment Theory*, London: Routledge.
5 Brown, G.W. and Harris, T. (1978) *Social Origins of Depression*, London: Tavistock Press.
6 Brown, G.W., Bifulco, A. and Andrews, B. (1990) 'Self-esteem and depression: 3. Aetiological issues', *Social Psychiatry and Psychiatric Epidemiology 25*: 235–243.
7 Bebbington, P.E., Hurry, J., Tennant, C., Strut, E. and Wing, J.K. (1981) 'Epidemiology of mental disorders in Camberwell', *Psychological Medicine 11*: 561–579.
8 Dr John Bowlby has been very influential in emphasising the importance of attachment in human development from a psychoanalytic basis. See for example the *Attachment and Loss* trilogy: vol. 1, *Attachment* (1969); vol. 2, *Separation, Anxiety and Anger* (1978) and vol. 3, *Loss, Sadness and Depression* (1980), Hogarth Press and the Institute of Psycho-Analysis. The books were republished in paperback by Penguin in 1978. An excellent summary of Bowlby's work is given in Holmes, J. (1993) op. cit. note 1.
9 There is a considerable body of published work by Professor Sir Michael Rutter and his team at the Institute of Psychiatry. Possibly the earliest to have impact was *Maternal Deprivation Reassessed* (1972 and 1981), Middlesex: Penguin Books.
   Recent publications include: Rutter, M. and Smith, D. (eds) (1995) *Psychosocial Disorders in Young People. Time Trends and Their Causes*, Chichester: Wiley and Sons.

10 Michael Rutter's research with David Quinton on the consequences of institutional care and intergenerational continuity has also been influential. For example: Quinton, D. and Rutter, M. (1984) 'Parents with children in care, II: intergenerational continuities', *Journal of Child Psychology and Psychiatry 25*: 231–250.

11 Proponents of 'false memory syndrome' include: Loftus, E. and Ketcham, K. (1994) *The Myth of Repressed Memory: False Memories and Allegations of Sexual Abuse,* New York: St Martin's Press.; Ofshe, R. and Watters, E. (1995) *Making Monsters: False Memory, Psychotherapy and Sexual Hysteria*, London: Andre Deutsch Ltd.

12 See for example Masson, J. (1984) *The Assault on Truth: Freud and Sexual Abuse*, London: Harper Collins.

13 The Present State Examination (PSE) was used to assess symptoms of depression. Wing, J.K., Cooper, J.E. and Sartorius, N. (1974) *The Description and Manual for the PSE and CATEGO System*, Cambridge: Cambridge University Press.

14 See for example, Beck, A.T. (1967) *Depression: Causes and Treatment*, Philadelphia: University of Pennsylvania Press.

Part I

Neglect

The next three chapters focus on failure to care for the child in terms of three related experiences. First, we assessed material neglect by parents. Second, we examined 'role-reversal' in which the parent abdicates responsibility for care, requiring the child to take on parental responsibilities and at times to provide care for the parent. Third, we considered emotional neglect in terms of 'antipathy' and rejection from parents. All three experiences tended to occur together in the same households. In particular material neglect proved fundamental as a basis for other forms of lack of care and abuse. Indeed, in case histories of material neglect it was common to simultaneously encounter descriptions reflecting the child's servant-like status in the home and the rejection and dislike shown by parents. This triad of experiences defined the uncaring family environment.

The experiences described exist at the extreme end of the continuum of behaviour exhibited by many parents. Most parents are inattentive to their children on occasion, expect them to contribute to household chores and are critical of their behaviour from time to time. These experiences are fairly innocuous at such a mild level. However, at more extreme levels these experiences are capable of causing long-term damage to children, despite being fairly prevalent in the community at large.

The effect of neglectful experiences are examined in terms of damage to the child's sense of self, relations to others and coping, as well as depression in adult life. Self-esteem in childhood was assessed by asking each woman whether she ever felt inferior to others, inadequate in terms of her appearance, personality or capabilities, and unpopular. We also questioned about the child's sense of self in relation to others in terms of feelings of shame about herself and her family with reference to home conditions, and how she felt these were viewed by the outside world. Finally we asked about loneliness in terms of being isolated and craving friendship and support. To assess coping, we asked whether the child had strategies for avoiding, ameliorating or halting adversity. This included help-seeking and strategies for escape, and planning for the future in terms of home leaving and future career. We assessed the lack of these as helplessness, particularly when accompanied by signs of defeat and hopelessness. The converse we assessed as good coping or mastery.

We sought to test whether neglectful treatment by parents restricted a child's ability to socialise, to develop a sense of self-worth and to see herself as an active agent in the world. A distortion of any of these developmental processes we considered likely to increase risk of disorder in adult life.

Chapter 2

Neglect: never truly available

For some the very existence of a caretaking and supportive figure is unknown; for others the whereabouts of such figures have been constantly uncertain. For many more the likelihood that a caretaking figure would respond in a supportive and protective way has been at best hazardous and at worst nil. When such people become adults it is hardly surprising that they have no confidence that a caretaking figure will ever be truly available and dependable. Through their eyes the world is seen as comfortless and unpredictable; and they respond by either shrinking from it or doing battle with it.

(Bowlby 1978: 242)[1]

All children need a basic modicum of care to survive. Without food, shelter and protection, they are unlikely to mature to adulthood. Extremes of neglect can lead to babies being abandoned on rubbish heaps or children dying through starvation and lack of medical care. Fortunately, these examples are fairly rare in our society. What occurs more often is pervasive neglect, shown by an absence of care and concern. This is a silent type of abuse often unnoticed or remarked upon by the outside world. Absence of care cannot be evidenced by physical scars, by violent acts or dramatic dangers. Neglected children typically *do* survive to adulthood but with various psychological handicaps, particularly those involving a sense of identity, self-worth and mastery.

Neglect itself is often neglected. The most recent NSPCC report, Childhood Matters, states that neglect, 'is not a problem which is perceived with the same severity as physical or sexual abuse . . . yet other forms of abuse are often accompanied by neglect . . . gross neglect can cause death or serious long-term damage'.[2] This is despite the fact that in 1996 over 9,000 children were *added* to child protection registers in England in a single year because of gross neglect.[3] Greater media attention has typically been directed toward the more dramatic instances of physical, sexual or psychological abuse. However, these abuses are often underpinned by a basic failure to recognise the child's needs for material and emotional care.

The following quote gives some indication of the way in which extreme parental neglect contains elements of repugnance towards the child: 'Neglected children learn to adapt to a lack of physical contact. They come to expect that their mother will not touch them, will seldom speak to them, and will ignore them for long periods of time. Such children may accommodate to this lack of nurturing by becoming sullen, withdrawn, and even hostile as they learn that the world is a cold, lonely and unfriendly place.'[4] Neglect such as this, conveyed by an avoidance of physical contact, was often spontaneously recounted in the childhood histories we collected. Statements such as: 'I didn't get picked up when I was a child in case I got spoilt' indicated how some parents withheld physical contact and affection as a matter of principle.

The earliest studies of neglect arose from investigations of maternal deprivation and loss. In extreme forms children were abandoned after losing a mother, whether to barren institutional settings or to haphazard care from adults with little commitment to the child. Early investigations into institutional care in the 1960s commented on the effects on children of receiving no human contact leading to a 'failure to thrive'. Such children became listless and apathetic even when adequately fed and clothed.[5] In more recent times television pictures of neglected children in Romanian orphanages in the chaos following the fall of the communist government showed similar behaviour. This focus on the experience of the loss of a mother meant that neglectful experiences were often not fully investigated in their own right, only as the aftermath of a mother's absence. Yet a mother or father may be present in the household but still neglectful of the children. As one woman in our series said about her mother, 'Even when she was there, she wasn't there.' There is one further practical feature of neglect. As well as involving distance and disregard from parent figures, it also involves the absence of a protector to shield the child from outside dangers. Through the experience of neglect, children are often left prey to other perils. When children are unsupervised they maybe injured whether by accident or through the actions of predatory adults or even peers. Thus neglect can be a magnet for other forms of trauma and disadvantage.

In addition to such practical dangers resulting from neglect, its psychological effects are also pervasive. A little girl's first point of reference to the world is through her parents, particularly her mother. Through this contact she learns to identify herself as an individual, learns to relate to the outside world and begins to explore and to learn from the security of that first relationship. When this relationship is characterised by neglect, disinterest and distaste the child can only conclude that she is unlovable and the world is hostile and unsafe. Consider the following definition by Jon Allen of the origins of self-esteem: 'Looking at others is like looking in to a mirror. You see the "me" in reflection. How you see yourself reflects how you are seen by others, how you are treated by them and how you feel in relation to them. Many persons have been told they are bad in myriad ways. But you need not be told directly; when you are mistreated you naturally conclude you are bad in some way.'[6] What is interesting about this statement is the comment 'you need not be told directly'. Neglect often involves rejection by implication, through lack of recognition and acknowledgement.

DEFINING NEGLECT

One of the reasons given for the failure to adequately identify child neglect nationally has been the problem of its definition. This has been considered somewhat vague in relation to other types of abuse, such that the level at which intervention is required is more open to interpretation. Definitions of neglect are necessarily framed in the negative: the reverse of the care that is required for healthy growth. Unlike other abuses one cannot describe the frequency with which certain acts occurred but rather the regularity with which certain things did *not* occur. Whereas abuse concerns the experience of a hostile or negative act, neglect involves the absence of a caring or positive act. It is a sin of omission rather than commission.

To assess parental neglect, we first considered what a child ideally needs for healthy growth and psychological well-being. Clearly material care is fundamental: being adequately fed and clothed, kept clean, given shelter and warmth and medical care if ill, are all essential to sustain life. In addition, emotional care is essential for psychological functioning. A child needs to feel protected and safe in the hands of observant and concerned adults. Encouragement of social contact through friends is necessary for the child to learn how to relate to others and acquire support. A child also needs to learn practical skills and to have a basic education in order to communicate well and cope with life's challenges. When these elements are present a child acquires a sense of social identity, self-worth and mastery over the environment. We decided that the absence of these conditions was indicative of neglect. Thus disinterest in material care, friendships, school work and the child's illness or distress were considered relevant for assessing neglectful parenting.

To enhance women's memory of the care given in their early years, we first asked questions about a 'typical' day in mid-childhood and obtained descriptions of family roles and routines. This was a fairly simple way of discovering what daily life was like for the child. Thus each woman was asked who had been responsible for waking her, making breakfast, taking her to school and so on throughout the day. We asked who provided meals, washed clothes and bathed her. The highest ratings of neglect tended to involve material neglect where children went hungry or cold. We asked whether parents took an interest in their friendships and encouraged them to bring friends home. We also asked whether parents protected them from known harm such as being bullied or isolated at school. In terms of school work, women were asked if parents checked that homework was done, read school reports, came to school open days or showed interest in the child's future employment. Finally it was ascertained whether the parents attended to the child personally in terms of offering emotional support or comfort when she was distressed or ill, and whether her birthday was celebrated and treats provided on other family occasions.

By assessing all this information we were able to assemble a picture of whether the parents were generally indifferent and neglectful. We thus questioned for factual information about daily routines, without letting the woman's *feelings* of rejection or bitterness influence our ratings. We only rated parental neglect as present where we had relevant concrete examples of incidents for which full details could be collected. It was fortunate that we took this approach since, as with other abusive experience, the negative accounts were often initially underplayed. It was only through careful and systematic questioning that the full story often emerged. We graded the accounts on a four-point scale reflecting the severity of the experience, with the highest point, 'marked', for the worst experiences of neglect followed by 'moderate', then 'mild' and finally 'little/none' where we judged none to be present. The following examples give an indication of how we defined these rating points.

'Marked' neglect

One woman recollected her bleak early childhood: 'You had the bare essentials, you had your bed, you had your wardrobe and that was it. You didn't have nice things in your room. Dad wouldn't let us have lights on in the bedroom, we'd have to do homework by the light of the TV. Dad slept most of the day because he worked nights. We maybe saw him when we were going to bed.' About her mother she said: 'If we came home from school there wouldn't be a meal on the table, she'd probably be asleep. She'd give us some money to go around and get a cake for our dinner, she used to feel school dinner was enough. I often went to bed feeling hungry. No one made breakfast – you did it yourself if there was any food there. Sometimes we'd oversleep and it was too late to have breakfast, so we'd just have to have a quick wash down and run up to school. We bathed ourselves, with two of us in the bath and we'd save the bath water for the others. Mum never washed our clothes, we took them round to the launderette. She used to keep me off school on a Friday to do all the shopping.' The woman recalled no instance of either parent being loving or supportive of her or caring for her when ill. She did, however, recall her mother (but not her father) remembering her birthdays, 'I would get a card, no party, but I might have a little tea among the family.' She also remembered a single outing with her mother when they went on holiday together without father. These few positive instances seemed more poignant given the indifferent context in which the child lived, and she treasured these moments as the only happy memories of her early years.

'Moderate' neglect

The next example is characterised by emotional coldness and disinterest more than absence of the basic necessities of life. This child was about ten when her mother left her in the custody of her father who sent her away to boarding school. Although the family were materially well off, she said, 'I always felt very deprived, particularly at boarding school. At Christmas I got nothing, no presents, no extra treats. My father never wrote to me or enquired how I was.' She returned home to her father in the holidays but found him cold and unapproachable. 'He would never kiss or hug me. In fact he never touched me.' She gave an instance of one night when she woke frightened. 'I had the most awful nightmare and woke up crying. He woke up and came in angry and shouted at me. I couldn't tell him anything. You were in fear of being found out, of unknown terrible things that might happen to you – life was always a cover up.' He never enquired about her life at school and knew nothing about her friendships. However, he was keen for her to do well academically and took some interest in her school work.

In this case the child's material needs were looked after and her father showed concern about her academic development. However, he was completely inattentive to any other of her other needs: when frightened he scolded her; at Christmas he sent her no presents; he never communicated with her or asked her how she felt. This was therefore rated lower than the first example which showed both material and emotional disinterest, but nevertheless was considered to be at least 'moderately' neglectful parenting.

'Mild' neglect

One woman suffered mild neglect from her father after her mother died when she was a baby. Her father brought her and her three siblings up single-handedly: 'He would work nights and be at home during the day and would always cook our evening meal. He didn't actually neglect me, I always had what the others had. But although I wasn't neglected materially, I was in terms of attention. I felt he never actually wanted me. My father knew who my friends were, there were lots of them in the street, he didn't mind me mixing with them. But he wasn't as interested in my school work because I didn't go to grammar school like my brothers and sister, although he did read my school reports. We never saw eye to eye. As long as I can remember we've never got on. He always tried to make me feel guilty. My father was a very hard man, you couldn't go to him if you were upset. He was never sympathetic.' Although there was tension between father and daughter, the child was adequately looked after in terms of her material needs. Thus 'mild' neglect reflected the father's unsympathetic attitude towards her emotional needs.

PREVALENCE OF NEGLECT

In our Representative London Women series we found 17 per cent had experienced parental neglect at a 'marked' or 'moderate' level.[7] This was measured in terms of absence of care from *both* parents. However, in practice the mothers' behaviour was particularly important since a caring mother often shielded the child from a neglectful father. The reverse proved to be rarer, with fathers typically less involved in household and childcare activities. We first came across experiences of neglect when exploring the ill-effects of losing a mother in childhood, and found neglect to be common as a consequence of such loss: 39 per cent of women suffered neglect associated with maternal loss compared with 10 per cent of those without such loss.[8, 9, 10] Among women who lost their mothers when they were little, the behaviour of stepmothers or other replacement mothers was particularly crucial in understanding the origins of neglect. We discovered, for example, that despite poignant accounts of the pain felt by the child at the death or separation from mother, it was the subsequent neglect from replacement parent figures that was related to longer-term damage. In particular, parental neglect was four times as common after the loss of a mother when a stepmother took over responsibility for childcare.[11] Closer investigation showed this was due to the presence of step-siblings or half-siblings resulting in large family size, with the father's children by his first marriage typically having lower status and less call on resources. These families were often in financial hardship which placed a strain on the second marriage leading to discord and marital problems.

The following example illustrates neglect from a stepmother after the child lost her mother from tuberculosis when she was a baby. Her father remarried when she was about four and she and her brother and sister moved in with him and their new stepmother and step-siblings. Two more children were soon born, resulting in seven children living in the household. Life became a struggle financially, and it was clear that the father's children from his first marriage had the lowest priority and took the burden of neglect. The woman recalls life with her new stepmother: 'She never fed me, I got very thin, I was sent away after a medical at school, to be fed. I wasn't allowed to sit and eat with them at the table. I used to have to stand in the corner. My sister, brother and I didn't have much to do with them, we were put into one room downstairs and they lived upstairs. Father was never there, he worked seven days a week. There was no family life for us at all. She favoured her own children. It was sort of like "us" and "them".'

However, not all stepmothers were indifferent to their stepdaughters. Some showed a good deal of care and patience with the children they had inherited from the new husband, as illustrated by the case of one woman whose mother died when she was nine and father remarried two years later. Although the child was rather rebellious, her new stepmother took good care of her, and established structure and security in the household. Her stepdaughter says of her: 'She had life, enthusiasm. She was great. She was ideal to bring children up. With my stepmother everybody had their job and at the end of the day you were so glad because you were capable of doing everything. There were certain standards, you wouldn't do anything to displease her.'

THE CONTEXT OF NEGLECT

There are many reasons why parents show indifference to their children. We observed that it often occurred when families were put under stress by circumstances such as maternal loss, financial strain, large family size and parental psychiatric disorder. It was not a particularly malicious abuse: children were ignored rather than beaten or exploited, their presence simply not accommodated or acknowledged. Although the family environments in which various forms of neglect and abuse arise will be discussed more fully in chapter eight, the following examples serve to set the scene for considering the wider family context of parental neglect.

Poverty

We did not consider poverty in itself to be an indicator of parental neglect. It was not the lack of resources we were assessing but the extent to which parents made sacrifices for the children and provided the utmost possible care within their financial means. Yet the two were closely linked. For example, at times acquiring money took priority and the children took second place. In the following family a woman reported how her parents were always working to make ends meet and provide for a large family: 'We would make our own breakfast or the older children would make it. We were brought up from a very young age to do things for ourselves. I started ironing when I was about nine years old and we were all responsible for washing clothes. Father would help in the home but mother didn't because she worked the longest hours. I was so quiet as a child, maybe because there were so many of us, I felt as if they didn't really have time for us. The only communication I ever had was at school or whoever I was sharing a bedroom with at the time. My mother hadn't really got time for me because she was always working. She didn't buy me things, like dollies. Sometimes I felt she wasn't really my mother because she was hardly ever around. I longed for grandparents to be close to, but I never knew any of them.'

Parental neglect was not an automatic consequence of poverty. In the following example the father's commitment to his children meant that they were cared for despite financial difficulties. This particular woman was brought up in rural Ireland with her five full-siblings and four half-siblings. Her mother died when she was seven and her father looked after the children, with the help of the eldest daughters. The family were not financially well off because the father was retired and living on a pension. However, they managed to survive and the children were well cared for despite the economic constraints. 'Those relatives that came over to England sent us home clothes. We had an aunty in America that was ever so good to us. She'd send us parcels.' Her father never considered putting the children into local authority care: 'I can remember one day daddy was digging in the garden and a neighbour came along and suggested putting us in a county home and father chased him up the road with a garden fork. Father spent all his time with us. He would always make sure we had enough to eat and there was somebody to look after us. It was him who cooked breakfast for us before we went to school. He'd sit and talk about mammy, and about when he was a boy. We really used to love it. He always cared about my school work. He couldn't understand why I didn't pass my scholarship. I think he was a bit disappointed. But he wouldn't send me to boarding school. He thought the nuns were too strict. He knew all my friends and if I wanted to go into town as a teenager he would arrange a lift for me. I'd give anything to go back to my childhood. We must have had our bad times but they were all sunny days.'

Parental psychiatric disorder

Some instances of parental neglect could be clearly traced to psychiatric disorder, particularly alcohol problems. Such disorder was associated with other family problems involving parental separations, financial hardship and discordant marriages. The following example shows how a parent's alcoholism (in this case the mother's) can have a detrimental effect on a child's care: 'One morning when dad come home from working nights, mum was so out of it with her hangover, I asked dad "What can we eat for breakfast?" and he said "There's bread and jam, you can have that." But there was absolutely nothing in the house for us to eat and we had to go hungry all day. Generally there was never anyone to make sure we were washed and tidy. My mum only had a bath herself every five to six months. It was terrible. She didn't like the house clean. Most of the clothes we had were given to us. Yet my parents did have money. The trouble was my mum used to waste it on drink and my father used to save it up for his retirement. Saving up for a rainy day.' Her parents were unavailable if she needed help: 'I got a nail through my foot once on Christmas day. I got up out of bed to see what I got from Santa and apparently I stepped on this nail. Dad put this great big dirty handkerchief around my foot. He never took me to hospital or anything. I walked around in pain for a week and when I went back to school they were very concerned. The school took care of it and got me antibiotics.'

In another case the father's drinking after his wife's death led to problems in the second marriage which had consequences for the child: 'They argued terribly. Then they wouldn't speak for a month. She lived in one room, he in another. They'd have meals at different times, she wouldn't cook for him or us, she wouldn't do the washing. It was his drinking that was the source of the problem. He got into debt. It caused a lot of unpleasantness. My stepmother was very moody. She would be nice one day and nasty the next. Like we had a big meal for Christmas day and then Boxing day she would refuse to cook and say, "get it yourself". She left home suddenly. I finished work one day, I was sixteen then and I was the first to get home. I opened the door and saw all the furniture had gone. She had taken everything. She'd left a kettle and two cracked cups for dad and me. She took literally everything. I suppose everything had to go for debts.'

CHILDHOOD SELF-ESTEEM AND RELATIONS WITH OTHERS

Women with parental neglect reported marked feelings of inferiority over twice as often in childhood as those who were well cared for.[12]

For example one such woman said: 'I didn't feel like everyone else. I felt my home life was too different. I was terribly shy. I felt inferior to the other children, so I kept myself to myself. I began to feel self-conscious about the way I looked when I was a bit older. I felt fat and that my sister was nicer looking and cleverer. I was never confident.' Neglected children also experienced greater help-lessness. In this example a girl's lack of confidence and timidity eventually came to affect her school work. 'I wouldn't put my hand up in class when I had a question or didn't understand something. It was difficult to ask for help from teachers and I never asked members of the family for help with personal problems. I didn't tell anyone when I became shortsighted. I couldn't see the black-board. I always felt inadequate in a lot of ways, especially in teenage years. I felt life happened to you, that you had no control over what happened.'

Since there was no one to facilitate social contact, and the children were rarely allowed to invite others to their homes, it was not surprising that the neglected children reported feeling lonely significantly more often.[13] One woman said: 'I often felt lonely. I spent most of my time by myself and I felt out of it. I felt things were going on without me. I kept a lot to myself because I found it difficult to make friends. I would go to school late, because I was shy and didn't have to talk to other pupils and also because I didn't feel settled.'

The children's isolation was sometimes due to feelings of shame about their families. This arose because the neglect was readily apparent to outsiders who witnessed their dirty clothes and houses and irregular meals. One woman commented: 'I felt ashamed about having a stepmother. I couldn't invite anyone back home. I felt self-conscious because I had no school uniform, I was the only one that wore an ordinary skirt not the school one. When she came up to school to see the headmistress everyone said she looked so severe. I never dared tell anyone what it was like at home.'

Another woman recounted how other school children noticed her change in appearance when she first came out of local authority care and was looked after by her stepmother: 'School kids told me afterwards, that they wondered about the great big car that came to pick us up after my mother's death – they thought we'd won some money. And then when we came back from the children's home, for the first couple of weeks they all thought we were really posh, because we had been given new clothes. I remember leaving the institution with two of every piece of clothing. A few weeks later, I remember wearing a terrible filthy, dirty dress, because it hadn't been washed properly. It was like in the books, literally like going down to rags. And the kids in school used to say, "What's the matter?" I can remember going to a girl's house after school and her mother almost crying, and taking the dress off me and washing it and drying it there and then.'

This example shows how stigma was associated with neglect, but it also shows how at times it elicited social support. Issues of protective factors will be discussed in a later chapter, but to anticipate the positive effects of support in childhood, an example will serve to illustrate its impact. The woman described earlier whose mother died of tuberculosis when she was a baby experienced support from two women during her childhood. The first was her next door neighbour: 'There was a couple next door. They had an older daughter and her bedroom was in the attic like mine. My stepmother used to lock me in the room and take the light bulb out. I was afraid of the dark, so I used to climb out of the window and sit on the roof. The woman next door used to come to her roof and tell me to come in and I would climb over.' An even greater intervention occurred when she was fifteen years old and had left school. Her school friend's mother, having heard how she was treated, let her come and live with her own family. 'I just left home one day for good and went to my friend's house. I didn't have anything to take with me, because I never owned anything. My friend's mother knew a bit about my background, but not all of it, I didn't sit and tell her everything. In fact she had confronted my stepmother about me before. In the end, after I left, the only way my father and stepmother could get me back was to get me made a ward of court. The probation officer came round to the family I was staying with to see how I was being looked after, and they said my father had no case. I was treated like one of the family. That's what I really liked about it.' Informal interventions such as these were not uncommon and were sometimes crucial for survival.

NEGLECT AND ADULT DEPRESSION

Neglect in childhood related to more than a doubling of rates of adult depression in each of the samples we studied.[14] For example in the Representative London Women series 34 per cent of those with either 'marked' or 'moderate' neglect in childhood were depressed in the year they were interviewed compared with 14 per cent of those with only 'mild' or no neglect.

THE EXPERIENCE OF SISTERS

As discussed in the last chapter, one complaint often raised against the use of childhood memory of experience to explain adult disorder is that the account of childhood may be biased either by poor recall or by exaggeration of past negative experience. We were therefore careful to collect factual information and question in sufficient detail to check for consistency in the accounts. We were also aware that it was necessary to check whether the childhood accounts were accurate. To do this we interviewed a 100 pairs of sisters raised together. Each sister in a pair was interviewed independently by a different interviewer and each was asked about her own and her sister's experience of neglect. From these independent 'double' ratings we were able to compare one sister's account of her own experience with her sister's corroboration. The level of agreement between the two would indicate the degree of accuracy in these accounts.

We found remarkably high agreement between sisters for the degree of neglect suffered, with 94 per cent of pairs agreeing about what had happened to each other.[15] We were also able to assess whether the sisters essentially had the same experience, or whether neglect was targeted more at one child in the family than another. We found the experience of neglect was largely shared by sisters, with 89 per cent having reported the same experience. [16, 17] Neglect, it appeared, was not personally directed but was rather a function of family characteristics typically affecting more than one, if not all the children in the family.

CONCLUSION

Neglect in childhood is a destructive experience inhibiting the child's capacity for physical and psychological development. The ordinary parental duties of feeding, washing and clothing the child are absent or mismanaged, as are the points of emotional contact through which the child can feel connected to its parent and so to the world. The child often interprets this personally and assumes she is unlovable and unworthy. The real reasons for neglect, however, appear to arise from the structure and characteristics of families. We know for example that it arises after the loss of a parent in the presence of step-parents, and where financial hardship and psychiatric disorder occur. Other circumstances may be involved too, and require further investigation before the full context of neglect can be understood.

We felt it important not to overlook parental neglect in assessing childhood experience. While the more dramatic abuses tend to reach newspaper headlines, neglect is just as damaging in both short- and long-term effects. The experience itself is pervasive and unalleviated. One cannot, for example, assess the frequency with which it occurs in the same way as is possible with physical or sexual abuse. Neglect in its most marked form happens all day, every day to children who are ignored and have their identity 'deleted'. Not surprisingly this is associated with low self-esteem and helplessness, features which often persist into adult life.

NOTES

1 Bowlby, J. (1978) *Attachment and Loss, vol. 2: Separation, Anxiety and Anger*, London: Penguin Books.
2 Report of the National Commission of Inquiry into the Prevention of Child Abuse (1996) *Childhood Matters*, vol. 1. *The report*, London: The Stationery Office.
3 NSPCC (1996) *Children and Young People on Child Protection Registers in England*, London: Government Statistics Office.
4 Webb, L.P. and Leehan, J. (1996) *Group Treatment for Adult Survivors of Abuse*, London: Sage Publications.
5 Rutter, M. (1981) *Maternal Deprivation Reassessed*, Middlesex: Penguin Books.
6 Allen, J. (1995) *Coping with Trauma*, Washington: American Psychiatric Press Inc.
7 In the Representative London Women series 17% (50/286) were rated as having either 'marked' or 'moderate' parental neglect.
8 *Table 2.1* Neglect and loss of mother (Representative London Women)

Loss of mother < 17	% with neglect (N)
Yes	39 (29/74)
No	10 (21/212)
	p < 0.001

9 Harris, T., Brown G.W. and Bifulco, A. (1986) 'Loss of parent in childhood and adult psychiatric disorder: the role of parental care', *Psychological Medicine 16*: 641–659.
10 Bifulco, A., Brown G.W. and Harris, T. (1987) 'Childhood loss of

parent, lack of adequate parental care and adult depression: a replication', *Journal of Affective Disorder 12*: 115–128.

11 In the Representative series, when *all* family structures lasting a year or more in childhood were investigated (N = 465, average of 1.61 per person) neglect occurred in 44% (12/27) of parent/step-parent arrangements versus 11% (49/438) of all others (p < 0.0001).

12 *Table 2.2* Neglect and childhood self-esteem and helplessness (Sisters series)

Neglect	% marked inferiority	% helpless
Present	28 (15/53)	34 (18/53)
Absent	12 (17/145)	12 (17/145)
	p < 0.025	p < 0.001

13 *Table 2.3* Neglect and childhood relations to others (Sisters series)

Neglect	% felt shame	% lonely
Present	68 (36/53)	58 (31/53)
Absent	34 (50/145)	31 (45/145)
	p < 0.001	p < 0.005

14 *Table 2.4* Neglect and adult depression in a 12-month period (% depressed)

Neglect	Representative London Women series	Loss of Mother series	Sisters series
Present	34 (17/50) .	37 (18/49)	40 (21/53)
Absent	14 (33/236)	10 (18/176)	19 (28/145)
	p < 0.001	p < 0.01	p < 0.025

15 Corroboration (accuracy in reporting on each other) of neglect in sister pairs was 0.70 (Kw, p < 0.0001) with 94% agreement in pairs.

16 Concordance (the degree to which they shared the neglectful experience) was 0.61 (Kw, p < 0.001), 89% agreement in pairs.

17 Bifulco, A., Brown, G.W., Lillie, A. and Jarvis, J. (1996) 'Memories of childhood neglect and abuse. Corroboration in a series of sisters', *Journal of Child Psychology and Psychiatry 38*: 365–374.

Chapter 3

Role-reversal: the meanest work of the house

'I'm twelve years old, please, sir, and my name is Margaret and I sweep a crossing in New Oxford Street. Mother's been dead these two years, sir, and father's a working cutler, sir; and I lives with him . . . Since Mother's been dead, I've had to mind my little brother and sister, so that I haven't been to school; but when I goes a crossing-sweeping I takes them along with me and they sits on the steps close by. If it's wet I have to stop at home, and look after them, for father depends on me looking after them. Sister's three and a half, sir, and brother's five.'

(Mayhew 1851: 408)[1]

Mayhew's account of the lives of costermongers in Victorian London describes how most working-class children at that time were expected to augment the family income by working. Very few received any education. Laws against child labour were introduced into the UK in the late 1800s although statistics from the last twenty years suggest that child labour is more common than might be expected and that rates in this country appear to be higher than in continental Europe.[2] Most of the children who work have been shown to be below the minimum legal age, a third doing prohibited jobs and an even higher proportion working illegal hours.[3] In addition to employment outside the home, recent estimates suggest that there are approximately 10,000 child carers working in the home, involving household duty and sibling care. A further 30,000 share such responsibilities with an adult.[4]

There are opposing views of the effect of children's employment, particularly when it occurs in mid-teenage years. On the one hand it is argued that children aged 14–16 can benefit from a certain degree of employment experience. Indeed many schools include 'work experience' for their older pupils. On the other hand it is argued that the combination of school work and employment can create over-tiredness in the child, cause a deterioration in school performance and create new dangers such as risk of accidents at work or in the home.[5] There has been little research establishing which of these suggested effects is the more likely outcome for the child.

The type of child labour we investigated in our study of women concerned the amount of work girls were expected to do in the home. That is, the extent to which they were used either as unpaid help, or as support for parents. The term 'role-reversal' refers to the switching of roles whereby the daughter takes over the parent's role and responsibilities. This can involve the daughter taking over the home-making role with responsibilities for cleaning, cooking and looking after younger siblings. It can also involve the daughter taking over an adult support role, acting as a confidant or counsellor for her distressed parent.

DEFINING ROLE-REVERSAL

In our series of women who lost their mothers when they were young, we measured the responsibilities imposed on the child in the household after the loss. We enquired about how much of the housework, sibling care or outside employment they took on after their mother's death. This dimension was further developed in the later study of sisters. We enquired not only about such practical responsibilities but also about emotional demands placed on the child, such as the parent depending on the child for confiding and comfort when distressed. We assessed the parent's helplessness in their parenting role and the child's concern and feelings of respon-sibility for the parent. From these different indicators we made a global rating of role-reversal. As with other childhood dimensions, we assessed the experience in terms of four scale points: 'marked', 'moderate', 'mild' and 'little/no' role-reversal before the age of seventeen.

'Marked' role-reversal

The following is an example of 'marked' role-reversal from a woman who was brought up by both natural parents. With ten children in the family her parents found it difficult to cope. There were heavy responsibilities imposed on the girl by her mother: 'I wouldn't say she was lazy but because there were enough of us to do what we had to in the house, she didn't have a lot to do. We did everything. I would be there in the morning, sending the other children off to school and I would check the house, I did feel like I was the mother. From nine onwards I was cooking and washing clothes and dressing the others. She didn't know how to cope with ten of us. I know that now. There were just too many of us. Mother couldn't cope with anything, certainly not a big family. *I* would be the parent. She always ran away from responsibility. When my younger sister had to see a child psychologist I was fifteen and mum said ''Go up to the school and sort it out, I'm not well.'' She was always complaining ''poor me'', always saying she was sick. I also had to keep secrets from my father. She'd say ''Don't tell him I've had a drink, that I've been in bed all day.'' My dad would sit and cry and cry, he never said why. He never confided in me, he always tried to cover things up. My father was sensitive and tried to hide his feelings.' She felt concern for both parents: 'I always worried they would die, worried that they would hurt themselves. I always checked the house for fear of fire. When they were fighting the only way I knew how to cheer them up was to sing and dance for them. Sometimes I would go and get them a drink to cheer them up.' In this instance it is clear that the daughter took responsibility for both running the household and for comforting and reassuring her parents, who were distracted by their marital problems. Parental neglect as described in the last chapter also permeated the situation.

'Moderate' role-reversal

Contrast the above example of 'marked' role-reversal with the following example rated as 'moderate' because of the largely emotional rather than practical support demanded. In this instance the mother lacked confidence and although able to cope with practical matters, was helpless in emotional ones. 'She was a very talented woman, a good manager. I mean she was a very able woman in many ways, but I sometimes felt that emotionally she wasn't. She confided in me first when I was nine. I don't remember feeling anything about it other than worried. I didn't think she shouldn't be telling me these things, even when I was little, because she was sad and she used to cry. She would tell me about how she felt. She made me feel guilty – told me she'd given everything up for us kids. I felt she needed looking after, I used to feel sorry for her. She would tell me she felt awful. I used to make cups of tea for her and try and see she was alright.'

'Mild' role-reversal

In the following example the child's mother was extremely moody and would stay in bed for days at a time. Her father took over much of the household responsibility with the help of his two daughters. However, since neither daughter was expected to take responsibility, only a 'mild' rating was made. 'When mother was out of action she would go to bed for two days and father would have to do everything, though he never took time off work. He'd expect me and my sister to do things as well. We didn't know what to do, we were all at a loss because we were never taught. We were told to do the washing up, but sometimes it was left. My mum didn't like us doing things. I don't know why. She had her own routine. I used to tidy the bedroom and my mother couldn't see why I wanted to do it. She could be very helpless. At times she wouldn't talk to anyone until she was able to cope.' Neither parent confided in the child, nor showed distress in front of her. In fact the girl had little sympathy for either parent.

PREVALENCE OF ROLE-REVERSAL

Our interest in role-reversal is comparatively recent and for this reason was not measured in the Representative London Women series. So although we do not know exactly how common it is in the community, we can make an approximate estimate from the later studies in which it was assessed. First, it rarely occurred without parental neglect, and second, between a third and a half of those with neglect were found to have role-reversal.[6] Thus since neglect in childhood occurred for 17 per cent of working-class mothers, then role-reversal is likely to be just over half as common, occurring in approximately 10 per cent of women at 'marked' or 'moderate' levels.

THE CONTEXT OF ROLE-REVERSAL

Role-reversal most commonly occurred in situations where the child also suffered parental neglect with rates ranging between a third and a half of those with neglect having role-reversal compared with between 10 and 18 per cent without. It was also more common after the loss of a mother: 60 per cent of women selected for early loss of mother had role-reversal as a consequence compared with 18 per cent without.[7] Role-reversal was most common in two sorts of family structure: first when father alone looked after the children and second when father and stepmother headed the household. The rate of role-reversal occurring in other arrangements was 17 per cent overall.[8]

Most of the role-reversal encountered in the accounts of the London women studied occurred in one of four different scenarios. The first followed the loss of mother, when the daughter herself stepped into the absent mother's shoes. The second scenario also occurred after such a loss but involved a step-parent forcing the child into servant-like status – the 'Cinderella' situation. The third scenario involved families where the mother could no longer cope for some reason and the child took the initiative and stepped into the breach. In the fourth situation the daughter was required to enter into a conspiracy with one parent against the other and tell lies on their behalf.

Daughter steps into absent mother's shoes

The experiences of the Victorian 'street-crossing' girl described earlier who had to work and look after younger siblings after her mother died bore many similarities with women we interviewed a century later. It was not uncommon for a girl in teenage years, or even younger, to be expected to take over the lost mother's role in running the household and looking after the younger siblings. Its association with neglect is illustrated in this next woman's story. Her mother died when she was thirteen. 'While Dad was at work I had to run the house, including cooking and washing. I didn't do the washing by hand, I sent it out to be done. My sisters didn't really help, they were too young. My father was working on night shifts. I sometimes didn't go to bed until 12 o'clock at night because of getting all the jobs done. I had to get Dad off to work at 9 p.m., then I had to look after the younger ones alone at night. The younger ones would squabble, I had to sort it out. Dad was home in the mornings and helped with breakfast.' She never missed time off school, but often arrived exhausted. Her father was capable but worked hard at his job and had little time to run the household. Despite the sorrow he felt at losing his wife, he tried not to show distress in front of the children. He became more anxious for their health because his wife died of cancer soon after youngest child was born. The girl never resented her role: 'I was pleased to be of use. I worried about him, he was so sad and missed mummy so much.'

The Cinderella situation

The famous fairy tale relates role-reversal by a stepmother: 'There was once upon a time, a gentleman who married for his second wife the most proudest and most haughty woman that was ever known . . . . He had by a former wife a young daughter of unparalleled goodness and sweetness of temper. . . . The stepmother could not bear the good qualities of this pretty girl . . . . She employed her in the meanest work of the house . . . she lay on top of the house in a garret. . . . When she had done her work she used to go into the chimney corner, and sit down upon the cinders.'[9]

A number of women spontaneously described themselves as 'Cinderella', being forced to do all the housework for their step-mothers while their step-siblings were given privileges. This involved a very different status from the first scenario described earlier in which the daughter effectively replaced her absent mother in terms of duty and status. In the Cinderella situation the daughter was also burdened with domestic responsibility but her status was subordinate to her new and often hostile stepmother. In effect she became an unpaid servant, almost as a compensation for the step-mother taking on her new husband's children. An example was given by a woman whose mother died when she was young. 'I used to do everything in the house. I was Cinderella. My sister and I used to do all the housework. I used to do all the washing, cleaning and cooking and the shopping. It started when I was nine. And I used to stick up for my younger sister. That made things worse for me. I was always the one up front who stuck up for the others. My dad had his own restaurant and I had to work in that as well, which I hated. So if he made me serve in the restaurant, I used to be rude to the customers. I stopped going to school. I just kind of dropped out. They complained at school. Of course I was kept off half the time to mind the younger children. Eventually the neigh-bours complained about how I was treated and I was put into local authority care for "my own care and protection".'

Parental helplessness: daughter as protector

Parental helplessness, particularly on the part of the mother, was often an important source of role-reversal. This sometimes resulted from mother's psychiatric disorder (such as depression or agoraphobia) or from her lack of skill (including an inability to organise, cook or look after numbers of children). Sometimes the mother's helplessness was a result of violent or controlling behaviour from her partner which at times also led to the child intervening to protect her.

In the following example role-reversal arose not only because of mother's nervous breakdown, but also because of her deafness: 'My sister was a "hole in the heart" baby. I was always made to feel watchful, from an early age, told not to wear her out, to look after her. I also had to look after a deaf and sick mother. Every knock on the door I had to tell mum, so I was parenting her too. I did a hell of a lot of housework, did all of it really. I first started aged eleven, ironing, washing the sheets. Mother couldn't cope with looking after herself, never mind us. We were able. But every now and then she would rally round. I felt responsible for her tears. I would worry about her mood swings. I felt unsafe because I was worried mum would die, especially after her first breakdown.'

A similar scenario emerged when a child tried to protect one parent from the other, typically the mother from the father's violence, as in this example: 'Mother never left the house because she would be frightened that dad would wreck it. She would normally just stand there and take any violence from him. She couldn't cope with dad, I felt that she used to sit around and not do a lot. She never really confided in me. She would cry and go into her room, never cry in front of people, but go behind closed doors. I worried about her, I felt it was my job to protect her. I was afraid dad would really hurt her. From the age of fourteen if he went into a rage I used to stick up for my mum. Then when he went mad, it was me that was in the line of attack.'

In the following family the daughter had to cope with the mother's psychiatric disorder and threats of suicide: 'I think she'd had enough and she didn't want to continue with us any more. She'd say to my sister who was a toddler, "Don't cry because you make mummy cry." She'd tell us she wanted to die. We had to hide her tablets from her. We had to hide the razor blades or turn the gas off so she couldn't gas herself. After my aunt died, mother always said she wanted to be dead with her sister.' The child's father often confided inappropriately: 'From the age of eleven, after my mother died, he started telling me everything he did, things he shouldn't have been telling me. Lots of stuff about his women friends and sexual stuff that I feel he should never have talked to me about.'

Keeping a secret

Occasionally the emotional role-reversal described above did not relate so much to the parent's helplessness, but to a parent drawing the child into a conspiracy against the other parent. Thus the role-reversal was of an emotional type whereby the child was confided in inappropriately and expected to collude with a deceit. Children were typically expected to keep secrets about extra-marital affairs or a parent's drinking habits. This put pressure on the children in a similar way to the 'helpless' parent, but involved greater manipulation of the child. We differentiated this type of secrecy from that imposed following abuse to the child herself, which is described in later chapters, and not included as role-reversal.

In the following example the mother confided in her daughter about her extra-marital affairs and made the child lie on her behalf to the father: 'I used to have to say she was out walking the dog. She told me I must never tell my dad. I don't know if the other children knew because I didn't mention it to anyone. If anybody got preferential treatment it was probably me, but only because she had to bribe me to do things, not to tell dad about her boyfriend.' This second example is similar: 'I had a secret with my mother which I had to keep from other people, which was about my father leaving her. The rest of the family didn't know it. They thought that my father worked abroad because of employment there, not because my parents had separated. I told my cousin about it when I was thirteen because I couldn't stand it any more, it was a secret just pressing down on me. She said, "You're going to go mad, go to a psychiatrist." In actual fact, the secrecy goes on to this day. I asked my mother about it again last year because my father who had been abroad, came back two years ago. I asked her "When exactly did he leave you" and she said, "Oh, when you were twenty-one, just before he went abroad." I wrote to him recently and said, "Please tell me when you left mum because I'm sure I've not been making this up all my life." He confirmed what I had always known. He said, "I left when you were about eight."'

'Women's work'

The issue of gender has not been discussed thus far since all our samples have been of women, and we have no descriptions of men's childhood experiences. However, from the women's accounts of role-reversal it appears that brothers were rarely expected to do similar amounts of work in the home. It was seen as the daughter's duty to fulfil the role when the mother was unable to. Occasionally the father stepped into the role, and more rarely the sons in the family. In many instances this was a source of resentment and interpreted as covert favouritism. In this account for instance, the girl's brother had a very different experience from her: 'My sister and I both had a lot of responsibility in the house, but my brother used to get away with it. Up to the age of eight or nine I was quite sort of happy with my brother and then suddenly I had to stay at home and help when my younger sister was born and I resented that.' Similarly: 'My sister and I both had to help a lot in the house. We took it in turns to do the housework. I felt I had too much to do. My brothers used to be lazy, they weren't expected to do anything.'

ROLE-REVERSAL AND SOCIAL LIFE

The feelings children had about themselves and in relation to others when experiencing role-reversal were similar to those associated with neglect: there were higher rates of shame about the family and higher rates of loneliness than those with no role-reversal.[10] This resulted in part from the lower rate of social contact allowed to girls who were expected to run the household and support helpless parents. The children often missed out on opportunities for social contacts because of their increased work at home. For example: 'When I started secondary school I wasn't allowed out in the evening. They'd all be going round to a friend's house to listen to records but I wasn't allowed to go, I had to go home. They didn't know why I had to go home, but I had to help with the housework and look after the younger sisters and things like that. It was the same at the weekend. I had to be up at the crack of dawn with my dad, doing the hand washing which included sheets, and helping with the housework and shopping. It was like having a little maid for them to do the housework, look after your sisters, do the shopping, do the washing, and somewhere in between make sure you get a little bit of sleep and go to school and get good grades. If you didn't get good grades you got punished for it.'

Another effect of role-reversal was interference with school work as children missed school because help was required at home: 'I used to skip lessons, not every week, but I was home more often in the afternoons after play-time. My stepmother shut her eyes to it and encouraged you to do it. She would say ''I'm glad you've come home, you cook the dinner, while I go up the road.'' At one time I had a phase of not going to school, just after I came out of the children's home. The school made an example of me, and they put me down from the top class to the bottom one, and I had to work my way up again. But my stepmother used to encourage me to stay at home because I had to mind the kids. I was quick learning, I used to borrow the other kids' books, copy it into mine, give them back and get top marks, so they never really knew.'

The pressure of so much responsibility at home, as well as at school, sometimes affected the children's health. The same woman described how she felt: 'The rows between my stepmother and dad were mainly over her not doing anything in the house. I felt I couldn't stand another row, so I would do the housework. I can remember being at school and suffering terrible headaches – they call it migraine now – I can remember literally banging my head against the wall with the pain. I didn't know what to do with myself, and I went into hospital eventually. And I remember coming out of the hospital to the house and before I did anything else, I had to clean the house from top to bottom, and literally scrub the floors. And I just broke down and cried in the evening and said I couldn't stand it any longer.'

ROLE-REVERSAL AND COPING

Taking on the parental role required initiative, energy and competence on the part of the child. Although imposed by a parent, it also required the child's willing participation. Many of the children who accepted the role had a highly developed sense of responsibility towards parents and younger siblings. There was a sense of duty involved in looking after the family and as in the quote from Mayhew's study of Victorian London, often a strong sense of protectiveness for younger siblings. Clearly characteristics of the child enabled role-reversal to occur: such children were 'pro-social', felt concern and compassion for parents and siblings and had the initiative to be able to take on this arduous role.

Unlike neglect, role-reversal was unrelated to feelings of inferiority in childhood but instead was associated with good coping or mastery. Some 38 per cent with role-reversal were judged to be good copers compared with 14 per cent without role-reversal.[11] It seems that the competence exhibited in household tasks extended to other areas of life, as this example shows: 'When I was fourteen, I was able to run both the house and the bed and breakfast business. I was very confident. I never had problems asking for help, but I rarely needed it. From very early on I wanted to be a Wren (women's navy), I even got information from the school recruitment office. Mother was very drunk and could be aggressive at times. I would ring Alcoholics Anonymous for help. When I was twelve there was one incident where a tradesman was in the house and he wanted to take pictures of me and then tried to touch me. I knew it wasn't right and I told the man to leave. I could cope on my own.'

The same evidence of coping can be seen in Mayhew's 'crossing-sweeper' described in the beginning quote. In the interview the girl goes on to say: 'The notion come into my head all of itself to sweep crossings, sir. As I used to go up Regent Street I used to see the men and women and boys and girls sweeping and the people give them money, so I thought I would do the same thing. That's how it came about. Just now the weather is so dry, I don't go to my crossing, but goes out singing . . . I only go sweeping in wet weather because then's the best time. I generally take about sixpence from about nine o'clock in the morning to four in the evening when I come home. I don't stop out at nights because father won't let me and I've got to be home to see to the baby. I can't tell whether I will always stop at sweeping, but I've no clothes so I can't get a situation; for though I'm small and young, yet I could do housework, such as cleaning' (Mayhew, 1851: 410, see note 1).

ROLE-REVERSAL AND ADULT DEPRESSION

Role-reversal was associated with adult depression. In the Sisters series 38 per cent with role-reversal were depressed in the year of interview compared with 20 per cent without.[12] However, the association was even clearer once the related but more common experience of neglect was taken into account.[13] While for those with neither neglect nor role-reversal only 14 per cent were depressed, for

those with either experience 41 per cent had depression. This illustrates how it is necessary to take more than one negative childhood
experience into account simultaneously to obtain an accurate picture
of the relationship between experiences and outcomes.

THE EXPERIENCE OF SISTERS

Corroboration by sisters was not assessed for role-reversal, but from
the Sisters series of interviews it was possible to examine the extent
to which both sisters had the same experience.[14] There was a modest
association between sisters for the shared experience of role-reversal,
with sisters having the same childhood experience in 76 per cent of
cases. However, this is a good degree lower than the 89 per cent
concordance for neglect and reflects the fact that often only one child
is given such responsibilities. However, the level of association is
also consistent with the case history examples which showed that the
role was often passed on when the elder girl left, or that more than
one daughter often shared the tasks. This was particularly where
responsibility for practical household tasks was concerned rather
than responsibility of an emotional nature. The following accounts
from a pair of sisters illustrate similar versions of the
'Cinderella' situation.

   The sisters were aged four and eight when their mother contracted
cancer. Both children were sent to a children's home until their
mother died. They then came back to live with their father. He
employed a housekeeper to live in and look after them. She brought
her young son with her and as time went on the housekeeper spent
more time looking after her own son and neglected the two girls.
The eldest sister recalls: 'It did start off quite well and then it sort of
got worse, which is natural. She favoured her son which caused
friction. We had to do most of the housework. You'd be cleaning
out the fireplace when you came home from school and lighting the
fire. I used to have to clean the stairs down, and make our beds, and
do our own linen. She often used to chase us round the house in
anger. We were lucky if we could get away. She used to pick on us
basically all the time. I resented it terribly, yeah, resented everything
there.'

   The younger of the sisters was only six when her mother died. She
reported feeling very unhappy with the housekeeper and recalls the
neglect both girls received: 'When I was very young I got on better
with her, and then I don't know if it's because her relationship with

my father got bad, but as we got older we had to do all the housework. She favoured her son tremendously and I think any resentment she held against my father she took out on my sister and I. We
basically ran that house. We did all the housework between us
completely. Even taking big heavy sacks of washing down to the
laundry. She went out to work in the end and we had to look after
her son in the school holidays.'

CONCLUSION

The effects of children being given responsibility in the home echo
the dilemma parents face in terms of protecting their children from
adult responsibility while also exposing their children to these
experiences in order to prepare them for later life. The message
from this chapter is clear: too much exposure, too young, accompanied by coercion and criticism from parents is damaging to mental
health. On the emotional side children are overburdened by having
to cope with their parents' weakness whether by inappropriate
confiding, preventing suicide attempts, protecting one parent from
the other or having to collude with family secrets. On the practical
side, when expected to help run the household and look after
younger siblings, children are denied crucial developmental experiences involving education and relationships due to the burden of
excessive domestic work. They feel alienated from other children
and have no time for normal childhood pursuits. Most perform the
role spurred on by concern for the younger siblings, anxiety about
the 'weak' parent, and a sense of responsibility for the family
staying together. Some feel deep resentment for being placed in
this position, particularly when they notice their brothers are
exempt. Adult workload and responsibilities come all too quickly
and last a long time. It seems little to ask for childhood to last for
at least sixteen years without these burdens.

NOTES

1   Mayhew, H. (1851) 'The girl crossing-sweeper sent out by her father',
    in P. Quenell (ed.) *Mayhew's London*, London: Spring Books.
2   Low Pay Unit Response, to Department of Health, *Employment of
    Children: A Consultation Document*, January 1996.
3   Pond, C. and Searle, A. (1991) *The Hidden Army: Children at Work in
    the 1990s*, London: Low Pay Unit.
4   Report of the National Commission of Inquiry into the Prevention of

Child Abuse (1996) *Childhood Matters*, vol. 1, *The Report*, London: The Stationery Office.
5 McKechnie, J., Lindsay, S. and Hobbs, S. (1996) 'Child employment: a neglected topic', *Psychologist 9*: 219–222.
6 *Table 3.1* Role-reversal and parental neglect (% role-reversal)

Neglect	Adult Risk series	Sisters series
Present	35 (13/37)	51 (27/53)
Absent	10 (7/68)	18 (26/145)
	p < 0.001	p < 0.001

7 *Table 3.2* Role-reversal and loss of mother (% role-reversal)

Loss of mother	Loss of Mother* series	Adult Risk series
Yes	60 (45/75)	31 (11/35)
No	18 (8/45)	13 (9/70)
	p < 0.001	p < 0.001

*Subsample of 120
8 *Table 3.3* Role-reversal and family structure (All household arrangements of at least 12 months reflected) (% role-reversal)

	Loss of Mother series (120 subsample)	Adult Risk series (146)	Total (266)
a. Both parents	18 (8/45)	17 (15/87)	18 (23/132)
b. Mother alone	–	17 (4/23)	17 (4/23)
c. Father alone	65 (17/26)	43 (3/8)	59 (20/34)
d. Father/ stepmother	72 (23/32)	0 (0/2)	68 (23/34)
e. Other	29 (5/17)	8 (2/26)	16 (7/43)

c and d versus rest p < 0.001
9 Opie, I. and Opie, P. (1980) *The Classic Fairy Tales*, London: Granada.
10 *Table 3.4* Role-reversal and relations with others (Sisters series)

Role-reversal	% felt shame	% loneliness
Present	64 (34/53)	55 (29/53)
Absent	35 (51/145)	32 (47/145)
	p < 0.001	p < 0.01

11 *Table 3.5* Role-reversal, coping and inferiority in childhood (Sisters series)

Role-reversal	% good coping	% felt inferiority
Present	38 (20/53)	58 (31/53)
Absent	14 (20/145)	50 (73/145)
	$p < 0.001$	NS

12 *Table 3.6* Role-reversal and adult depression (Sisters series)

Role-reversal	% depressed
Present	38 (20/53)
Absent	20 (29/145)
	$p < 0.05$

13 *Table 3.7* Role-reversal, neglect and depression (Sisters series) (% depressed)

| Role-reversal | Neglect | |
	Present	Absent
Present	33 (9/27)	42 (11/26)
Absent	46 (12/26)	14 (17/119)
	NS	$p < 0.005$

14 Concordance of sisters' experience of role-reversal was 0.28 (Kw, $p < 0.01$) with 76% agreement in pairs. No figures are available for corroboration.

Chapter 4

Antipathy: ceaseless reprimand

Am I a servant? No, you are less than a servant for you do nothing for your keep. There, sit down and think over your wickedness. Why could I never please? Why was it useless to try to win anyone's favour? . . . I dared commit no fault: I strove to fulfil every duty; and I was termed naughty and tiresome, sullen and sneaking from morning to noon and from noon to night.

(Brontë 1847: 18) [1]

It has been suggested that for healthy psychological development children need at least one adult who is irrationally enthusiastic about them.[2] In most cases this unconditional affection is provided by a parent. Sadly, however, a significant number of children are made to feel that their parents endure them rather than enjoy them. While for some this is conveyed by a simple absence of parental affection and warmth, for others the situation is considerably more grave. Their childhoods are characterised by the presence of antipathy – an active loathing and rejection on the part of their parents. Estimates of the number of children in the United Kingdom who are raised in such hostile environments each year are as high as 350,000.[3]

Parental antipathy can show itself in a number of ways, as illustrated in Charlotte Bronte's *Jane Eyre*. Her poignant account of antipathy is now over a hundred years old, but little different from contemporary accounts. The opening pages of the novel recount how the orphan Jane was taken in by the Reed family who subjected her to 'a life of ceaseless reprimand'. While Mrs Reed's own children enjoyed all the comforts of home, Jane was detained in a bare room with no heating or food as punishment for what was perceived as her wickedness. Among our samples we found that marginalising a child by differentially apportioning resources between siblings was just one of the many tactics parents used to underline their hostility towards the child. Another was criticism, usually unwarranted and personal, attacking the appearance or personality of the child. These were the types of experiences we questioned about when assessing antipathy.

DEFINING ANTIPATHY

To qualify for a rating of antipathy, subjective feelings of having been unloved or disliked were insufficient. Claims of hostile parenting had to be substantiated by examples of critical and rejecting verbal and non-verbal behaviour directed at the child by the parent. Indicators of antipathy included constant criticism, parents being difficult to please and describing the child as a nuisance or burden, open favouritism of a sibling or scapegoating of the child, and withholding resources from the child in a differential way. It was also necessary to have evidence that such critical and rejecting comments or behaviour had occurred over a period of time and did not reflect a single occasion. Consistent with our other measures, examples of antipathy were graded in terms of severity ranging from 'marked' through 'moderate' to 'mild' and 'little/none', and rated separately for mother and father figures.

'Marked' antipathy

The following example was considered 'marked' because of the unrelenting nature of the criticism, unrelieved by periods of affection or concern for the child: 'I was constantly told I might be a bad example and that I'd led the other children astray. I was always very much to blame for anything that went wrong. I don't think any of us had proper attention or affection. Once when I sat down under a shelf I accidentally pulled the telephone cord that was hanging down and the phone fell on my head. It cracked my head really hard. I started crying. My mother just screamed and shouted at me. She said ''Pity it didn't crack your skull'' or something like that. During my adolescence she used to tell me I looked like a tramp – I looked like a whore. She said I might as well be on the streets.' In addition to harsh criticism, her mother was also particularly difficult to please: 'I took my parents breakfast in bed when I was aged four or five. By the time they got the toast it was cold. ''That was no good'' mother said. That was typical of her attitude towards me.'

'Moderate' antipathy

A 'moderate' level of antipathy embodied less vehement and pervasive criticism. This woman recalls: 'I can't remember playing games with mother. All I can remember her doing is telling me to go away and leave her alone: ''Go and play on your own'' or ''Go and play with your sister.'' She was never positive about me. If I had achieved something at school, she never actually praised me for achieving something, it was no more than she'd expected. But if I failed she'd never let that go. She'd complain for weeks that I wasn't good enough. She'd say I wasn't a very nice sort of person – why wouldn't I be nice? If I tried to help, she wasn't satisfied. I didn't argue with her because I realised you couldn't get anywhere with her.'

'Mild' antipathy

Examples of low-level antipathy involved a much milder form of parental criticism. Sometimes it took the form of infrequent comments confined to only one aspect of the child's behaviour, as this example demonstrates: 'It wasn't really dislike, it was just that father saw me as a projection of himself when it came to school work. He didn't see me as an individual person at all. He was impossible to please over school reports. If I got a good report then the teacher was an idiot, and if I got a bad report then I wasn't really trying hard enough. It was impossible to get it right.' Yet in other respects her father was tolerant and affectionate.

NON-VERBAL ANTIPATHY

Although antipathy was often shown verbally, it could also be indicated by non-verbal behaviour. This was demonstrated in the case of a woman whose father showed a total lack of love or concern for any of his children by use of exceedingly unreasonable behaviour. He was a heavy drinker who had worked as a painter and decorator but lost his job when the excessive shake in his hands – the result of many years of alcohol abuse – rendered him unfit to work. Reduced to surviving on state benefit, he often turned to the children to finance his drink habit. The woman recounted the lengths he would go to in extorting money from them: 'I used to do a paper round when I was about twelve and dad used to say to me "If you don't give me the £2 from your paper round for Guinness I'll take the plug off the iron", and stupid things like that. Or else we wouldn't be able to watch television until we'd given him whatever money we had. Then he got a slot meter television you had to put 50 pences in, and 50 pence was a lot of money in those days. So we'd put our 50 pence in so that we could watch "Coronation Street", but instead he'd switch over and watch what he wanted. Then at the end of three months when the money was emptied out of the slot machine, he'd get a rebate and keep the money and get drunk on it.'

SIBLING FAVOURITISM

Tactics employed by parents to ostracise the disliked child often included scapegoating and favouritism of others. Frequently one child alone was regarded as culpable for anything that went wrong: 'I got the blame for everything, from the washing-up not being done to mother having a heart attack.' We heard many stories of siblings being allocated more clothes, food, toys and presents, and being disciplined more liberally than the child in question. Gender was one reason for this differential treatment, with sons being favoured in some families. One woman described how her brother was sent to boarding school and avoided all the hostility in the household: 'He wasn't an ordinary family member, because of being sent to board- ing school. The "blue-eyed boy" we used to call him. He was mum's pet. Oh Christ, you should have seen the size of the boxes full of biscuits and shortbread she'd send to him every couple of weeks. And he'd get pocket money sent to him – pocket money! God! We didn't know what it was! He'd come home for his holidays and could do no wrong. He hadn't seen the criticism, arguing and hitting that was going on.'

Another fairly extreme example of such differential treatment of siblings was that of a woman who experienced material hardship even though she grew up in a relatively affluent family. Her parents considered her inferior because she was female. They told her repeatedly that they preferred sons. 'I was two when my brother was born and I was totally rejected after that. Whenever there was any conflict with him, I was always blamed. If he smashed my toys I wouldn't be allowed to cry or complain. When I tried to stand up for myself I'd be beaten. My father would criticise me. He would say that I was not worthy to be his daughter. I don't think he's ever been proud of me. I spent a lot of time avoiding my father, a lot of time wishing he was dead. I used to see other children sitting on their father's knee and think ''why can't my father show me love?'' He's intolerant of females, always blaming females.' There were striking differences in the way the son and daughter were treated. Brand new clothes were provided for the son while the daughter was dressed in clothes bought from second-hand shops, including her shoes, which were ill-fitting and resulted in her feet being covered in corns. Her social and educational development were marred too. She was never allowed out to play with other children, nor was she allowed to bring friends home. Meanwhile, her brother was allowed to socialise as much as he pleased. When her brother left school he was encouraged to study for college and was later set up in a business financed by their father. By contrast, the parents forced their daughter to leave school without taking exams. She received no help from them in finding employment, and drifted from one dead-end job to another for many years.

In the following example one child was scapegoated by both parents for no reason other than to compensate for being the father's natural child rather than his stepdaughter. She was also scapegoated because she wet the bed until teenage years due to a chronic kidney complaint which was never recognised by her parents. 'I think my father spent his life proving that I wasn't his favourite and my mum spent her life feeling that I was. Maybe I was his favourite in some sense, but he always tried to be hard on me, so the others wouldn't say he treated me any better. My mother always picked on me. She would tell my brother and sister not to play with me and not to talk to me at the dinner table because I was dad's pet. I've often asked my mother if she loved me and she's told me ''no''. She used to tell me I was dirty and scruffy. I was generally a disappointment to them, with all the bed-wetting. As a child, my mother favoured my sister, right up until she was about eighteen. She did more things with her. For instance, one year when my sister was doing well at school, she bought her a ring. If I'd done anything well at school she wouldn't have bought me anything. Mum bought her a new bra when she was first wanting to wear a bra. There was no interest when I needed one.'

Being a stepchild often led to more ostracisation. The case history covered in earlier chapters of the girl whose mother died of tuberculosis and was subsequently looked after by her neglectful father and stepmother illustrates this well. She was treated as inferior to her step-siblings, being forced to play and eat separately: 'When my father wasn't there I wasn't allowed to sit with them at table, I used to have to stand in the corner. When my father was home I was allowed to sit at the table. I don't think he knew, I was too afraid to tell him. I wasn't allowed to speak to my stepbrothers and sisters. Only if I had to look after them. You could never please my stepmother, no matter what you did. We weren't allowed to speak. We had to call her ''madam'', I never called her mother. She never showed any affection, any interest. She only complained and criticised.'

VERBAL ANTIPATHY

In addition to the non-verbal tactics of scapegoating and sibling favouritism, verbal displays of parental antipathy were common. Verbal assaults served to demoralise the child and crush any sense of self-worth. One woman, for example, was repeatedly referred to by her mother as 'that stupid bitch' throughout childhood. To add to the humiliation these put-downs were often expressed in public. Other remarks included parents telling their children they wished they had never been born, or even more aggressively, wishing them dead. This taunt posed a terrifying threat in the context of a violent home where such an outcome was indeed a possibility.

INTRUSIVE AND CONTROLLING ANTIPATHY

In contrast to such criticism based on lack of concern, some hostile criticism directed at children was derived from over-involvement. This type of hostility frequently showed itself in parents who placed unrealistic expectations on the child. Thus, with impossibly high standards of behaviour to maintain, the child inevitably failed to reach the goal they had been set and would be harshly criticised. One woman described how, as a child, she had sobbed her heart out in the school toilets because she was afraid to go home and tell her father, a school teacher, that she had scored ninety-nine out of a hundred in her maths exam. Despite being top of the class, she knew she would be severely reprimanded for failing to achieve 100 per cent. Her father's disparaging remarks guaranteed that she would never feel pride in her accomplishments. This sense of failure haunted her into her adult life: despite dazzling career achievements she was continually plagued by self-criticism and doubt.

Some women only experienced parental antipathy as they became teenagers and needed to assert their independence, as this woman described: 'When I was young it was different. She would cuddle, sit me on her knee and say she loved me. But as I got older she stopped being close. When I was fourteen I felt she didn't like me very much, but she didn't really reject me. When I had bad spots she would always go on about them. You don't want your mother to discuss your spots in company as a teenager! From about 14 there were a lot more restrictions – "You can't do this and you can't do that." Everything I did I felt was wrong. I was embarrassed about showing feelings towards my mother. Her strictness about times to come in used to drive me mad. I used to feel she wanted to know too much. She was very good at poking around in my things. You couldn't hide anything anywhere, she would find it. She'd say "Anything in this house is my business." She'd found sanitary towels in the room I shared with my sister that she thought were mine and started quizzing me about my periods. She could have just asked me outright without all that rigmarole. She liked having a look in drawers just to make sure she knew what we were up to.'

The same woman's father was also hostile towards her in teenage years. 'They were both hard to please and the two of them used to gang up on me. My father had always wanted a son. I don't think he knew how to handle girls, he didn't know how to talk to them. He wasn't all that interested. When I was a teenager he started getting worse. He would say, "This is my house and if you don't like it you can get out." He found me a nuisance. He felt he could open my mail if he wanted. If my parents suspected something was going on they would do that. I had a boyfriend when I was fourteen and he was a Catholic. My dad told me I wasn't allowed to go out with Catholics so I had to finish with him. My father hated the idea of any man coming near me. Nobody was good enough for us as boy-friends. He was very protective that way.'

PREVALENCE OF ANTIPATHY

In our Representative London Women series as many as 33 per cent of women experienced antipathy from at least one of their parents in childhood at a 'marked' or 'moderate' level.[4] But antipathy from both parents simultaneously, as in the above example, was relatively uncommon, reported by only 5 per cent. Antipathy from mother or mother-figure was highly related to loss of mother. In such cases the antipathy came from either a substitute mother who resented having to look after the child following the loss of natural mother, or else from a hostile natural mother prior to her leaving the child. In the Representative series 32 per cent with loss or separation from mother had antipathy from mother-figure compared with 12 per cent with no maternal loss or separation. Antipathy from father was unrelated to loss of mother.[5]

THE CONTEXT OF ANTIPATHY

Antipathy was more common among neglected children: 42 per cent of those with neglectful parents suffered antipathy from mother compared with 12 per cent of those without neglect. Figures for father were similar.[6] Results from the Adult Risk series showed that antipathy from mother but not father was associated with role-reversal. Over half of those with role-reversal also had antipathy from mother compared with 26 per cent of those without role-reversal.[7] There was no significant difference in rates of antipathy in different family arrangements.[8]

Sometimes dislike and hostility in the parent–child relationship stemmed from difficulties the parent experienced in controlling the child. In this context parents used criticism and rejection as a means of correcting undesirable behaviour, ranging from toddlers' tantrums to teenage rebellions. Often antipathy was viewed by parents not only as a necessary means of control, but also as ultimately beneficial for the child. It seemed these parents lacking any concern or empathy saw themselves as entirely justified in their hostile approach to child-rearing. One of the disturbing aspects of the maltreatment of Brontë's heroine Jane Eyre, for example, was Mrs Reed's justification for her own conduct. She claimed it was carried out with the child's interests at heart, declaring that, 'children must be corrected for their faults'. Some particularly severe instances of antipathy often had a sadistic undertone, and a number of such examples qualified as instances of psychological abuse, discussed in a later chapter.

Often the source of the parent's antipathy lay outside the child's behaviour. Struggling to cope with adverse circumstances such as unemployment or stressful work, financial hardship or poor housing – and not least the parent's own psychiatric disorder – took its toll on the amount of patience and understanding parents had left for their children. Some parents simply seemed worn down by the burden of caring for their children, as one woman commented: 'When mum got wound up she openly used to say: "I'll be better off when I'm six feet under." I think she resented us all, that she was lumbered with these four kids. I felt I couldn't do anything to please her. She was always moaning at us.'

Another factor that fuelled parents' hostility towards their children was problems within the parents' marriage. Irritability and tension between parents spilt over into their day-to-day interaction with the children, who became casualties of the marital war. Discord between parents was particularly common among those with antipathy from the father. Around a third of women (36 per cent) from discordant families also had antipathy from father compared with 14 per cent from non-discordant families. Similar figures held for antipathy from mother.[9] One woman clearly linked the disintegration of the parents' marriage with a deterioration in her relationship with her parents. She describes the mounting tension between her parents: 'Their personalities didn't work well together. It started with slamming doors and then they worked up to throwing each other around the room. They were *very* violent. I remember my mother going into hospital with broken arms and things.'

The same woman felt growing hostility directed at her by both parents for some time prior to her parent's divorce, and its development seemed to parallel the growth of problems within the marriage. Both parents showed irritability and impatience towards her: 'I remember them not treating me very well. I don't think they were pleased to have me around. I remember them losing their temper with me a lot.' Her parents finally divorced when she was thirteen, and she lived with her father. However, the hostility continued. As she grew, her physical similarity to her mother was a constant reminder to her father of his ex-wife, and in arguments with her father he would criticise her: 'You're just like your mother.' She felt like a thorn in his side, and left home as soon as she was old enough to get a job.

CHILDHOOD COPING AND RELATIONS WITH OTHERS

Children who suffered antipathy were at times rendered powerless, with no means of redress, as any protest they raised against their treatment was seen as insolent. This was typically viewed by parents as yet another character fault which had to be ironed out by further punishment. Women who experienced antipathy in childhood reported high levels of helplessness as children but this was most marked when the antipathy occurred from *both* parents. Some 41 per cent of women who experienced antipathy from both parents were judged helpless in childhood compared with 15 per cent who did not experience antipathy.[10] As with neglect and role-reversal, women reported higher feelings of shame and loneliness. Again this was most marked when the antipathy was from both parents, among whom three-quarters reported shame and loneliness compared with just over a third of other children.[11]

One woman who was continually told how inadequate she was by her parents expressed helplessness and pessimism about any influence she could have as a child over her life. These feelings extended into teenage years: 'I lacked confidence and I gave up too easily. My parents said my sister was cleverer than me and I believed it and just gave up. I didn't try to prove my parents wrong. I just assumed that was the case. I didn't try hard enough, I could have done much better at school if I'd tried a bit harder. I never stuck up for myself. I was always a loner. I didn't laugh much and I was probably a bit of a misery. I was always afraid of the world. I didn't make much of an effort to change my situation and I never felt confident. Things would seem to pass me by. But I was a capable child and I thought that as soon as I left school I would leave home. My friend was living in a house where there was a room if I wanted it. I arranged to move away from home and my dad helped me move. A week after I left school too. But that evening I decided that it was too much and I wouldn't be able to cope with leaving school and home in the same week, so I moved all my stuff back home. I gave up yet again.'

Some children's response to criticism was to struggle even harder to please their parents. One woman describes how she took on responsibility for much of the housework from an early age in the misguided belief that this would please her hostile mother. Her efforts were in vain, for the criticism continued: 'I dusted for her, I hoovered for her, I cleaned for her. Every week I would do it for her and still she wasn't happy with me. Whatever you did, you couldn't make her happy.' It didn't matter how much the child tried to make amends and be a 'good girl', the parent's criticism continued, relentlessly. Furthermore, complete obedience by the child at times reinforced the parent's controlling behaviour rather than raising their level of respect for the child.

Another woman whose mother was very hostile expressed her feelings about such treatment: 'I felt very self-conscious if I asked for help. I thought I'd get shouted at. Once I'd missed the driver who car-pooled us to school everyday and I got lost walking home. I hid in the toilet after coming back to my house because I was too embarrassed to ask my mum to drive me to school since I had missed my ride. I was also dominated by my sister. I felt like a *slave* to her. I couldn't stand up to her bossing me. I always did everything she told me. I was very timid and shy and I had a speech problem and because my sister used to do *all* the talking, she used to reply for me.' Sometimes feelings of powerless led children to pray for help. One woman recounted: 'I used to pray that my dad would die, that he would be killed at work, or that somebody would kill him in the pub, that he'd get into a row and somebody would kill him. I really meant that sincerely.' Not surprisingly, after years of criticism some children reacted with anger towards their rejecting parents: 'I hated mother with a passion. I wanted her dead. I used to take delight in not telling her things.'

While parents' hostility sometimes aroused anger and retaliation in the child, at times the child's hostility fuelled antipathy from the parent, and a vicious cycle was set in motion. Some children had hated their parents for as long as they could remember: 'I was told I was born prematurely. Do you know why that was? Because I must have thought (as a foetus) "I want to get out of here – I don't like her much!" I never really enjoyed being with my mother. Later I got to hate her. I loathed her. I felt disgust.' The task of untangling who initiated the antipathy between parent and child was one which we did not tackle. What we were primarily concerned with was measuring the quality of parenting impinging on the child, rather than who instigated the problematic parent–child relationship. In most cases, however, it appeared to us that the parent was the instigator of the hostility which emerged from the child's earliest years. Care was taken in distinguishing at least the direction of the hostility, even if not who initiated it, and we measured hostility expressed by the child towards the parent separately.

ANTIPATHY AND ADULT DEPRESSION

Although the experience of antipathy from either parent in childhood led to an increase in depression in adulthood, it proved to be the combination of antipathy from *both* parents which was responsible for the association: 54 per cent of women with this experience were depressed in the year of interview compared with 16 per cent of the remainder.[12] It would seem therefore that the presence of a positive input from one caring adult, or at least the absence of malice from that adult, may buffer some of the damaging effects of hostile treatment from the other parent.

THE EXPERIENCE OF SISTERS

Sisters tended to report different experiences of maternal antipathy. Some 67 per cent of pairs had similar treatment, substantially less than the 89 per cent for neglect.[13] From the case histories covered it appeared that one sister was often picked on more by the mother than the other. Yet antipathy from father was more likely to be similar for both sisters, with 88 per cent experiencing the same level of antipathy. However, the corroboration from sister to sister was still good, with 75 per cent agreeing on how the mother treated each of them and 89 per cent agreeing on father's behaviour.[14] This indicates that despite differences in the way they were treated, women were able to report accurately on their childhood experience.

The following example shows how although sisters might be treated differently they were still able to agree on the scapegoating of one and favouring of the other. It is the case described earlier of the woman picked on by her mother for supposedly being her father's favourite and for chronic bed-wetting. This is the account given by her sister, the mother's favourite, which showed great similarities with the account the woman herself gave: 'My mother and sister never got on. They argued a lot or they just didn't speak. My mother never liked her. They just didn't get on. From when she was six Mum told her she had to protect me and my brother and if any child touched us she should beat them up. She would get in trouble with my parents if she didn't do it and they would give her a smack. She was hit with a stick from when she was nine. She got picked on a lot. She would just get a good smack for wetting the bed. My mother would say my sister was jealous of me and my brother and that's why she wet the bed. The doctor explained that it was a kidney complaint but they still couldn't accept it, that she couldn't control it. There was no affection for her because dad had to prove she wasn't his favourite. He was harder on her, but she was still his favourite. He didn't show it, but you could just tell she was something special in his eyes. She had it harder than me because of my mother.'

CONCLUSION

One of the outcomes of healthy childhood development is the establishment of feelings of self-worth. A child needs the love and respect of a parent figure in order to let these feelings develop. Thus within this intimate relationship the parent has the power to germinate the child's sense of competence, dignity and self-confidence. By the same token, the parent has the power to thwart the development of these qualities in the child. This is precisely what happens in situations of hostile parenting. Such children become helpless, unable to please and appease. In the long term they are highly likely to experience depression: as many as half of women who suffered antipathy from both parents developed depression in the year we studied them.

As with neglect and role-reversal described in the previous chapters, antipathy is a form of child maltreatment which is rarely drawn to the public's attention. Despite its potential for long-term damage, it seems that the more dramatic forms of maltreatment such as physical and sexual abuse are more frequently the topic of media concern. While the latter forms of abuse are highly damaging, we hope to see increasing public awareness of the dangers of the lack of care shown to children in terms of neglect, role-reversal and antipathy.

NOTES

1 Brontë, C. (1847) *Jane Eyre*, London: Collins Clear Type Press.
2 Bronfenbrenner, U. (1978) 'Who needs parent education?' *Teachers College Record 79*: 773–774.
3 HMSO (1995) *Child Protection: Messages from Research*, London: HMSO.
4 Antipathy from mother at 'marked' or 'moderate' level occurred for 17% (50/286) and from father for 20% (56/286) of the Representative London Women with 33% (93/286) with antipathy from either. Only a small group of 5% (13/286) simultaneously had this level of antipathy from both parents.

5 *Table 4.1* Antipathy and loss of mother (Representative London Women series)

Loss of mother	% antipathy from mother	% antipathy from father
Yes	32 (24/76)	25 (19/76)
No	12 (26/210)	17 (37/210)
	p < 0.001	NS

6 In the Representative London Women series 42% (21/50) of those with neglect also suffered antipathy from mother compared with 12% (29/236) without neglect (p < 0.001). The figures for antipathy from father were 34% (17/50) versus 17% (29/236) respectively (p < 0.01).

7 *Table 4.2* Antipathy and role-reversal (Adult Risk series)

Role-reversal	% antipathy from mother	% antipathy from father
Present	55 (11/20)	35 (7/20)
Absent	26 (22/85)	21 (18/85)
	p < 0.025	NS

8 *Table 4.3* Antipathy from mother in different family structures (Adult Risk series: all family structures 12 months or more, N = 145)

Child living with	% antipathy from mother	% antipathy from father
a. Both parents	28 (25/88)	24 (21/88)
b. Mother alone	32 (8/25)	–
c. Father alone	–	33 (3/9)
d. Parent/ step-parent*	53 (9/17)	29 (5/17)
e. Other	7 (1/14)	0 (0/14)

* All but two arrangements were mother with stepfather

9 *Table 4.4* Antipathy and family discord (Representative London Women series)

Discord	% antipathy from mother	% antipathy from father
Present	27 (20/75)	36 (27/75)
Absent	14 (30/211)	14 (29/211)
	p < 0.025	p < 0.005

10 *Table 4.5* Antipathy from both parents and the child's helplessness (Sisters series)

Antipathy from both parents	% helplessness
Present	41 (7/17)
Absent	15 (28/181)
	p < 0.001

11 *Table 4.6* Antipathy from both parents and the child's relations to others (Sisters series)

Antipathy from both parents	% felt shame	% loneliness
Present	76 (13/17)	76 (13/17)
Absent	40 (73/181)	35 (63/181)
	p < 0.01	p < 0.01

12 *Table 4.7* Antipathy and adult depression (% depression)

Antipathy from	Representative London Women series	Adult Risk series
a. Both parents	54 (7/13)	69 (9/13)
b. Mother only	16 (6/37)	45 (9/20)
c. Father only	26 (11/43)	25 (3/12)
d. Neither	13 (26/193)	30 (18/60)
a vs rest	p < 0.001	p < 0.025

13 The correlation between sisters for having had similar experience of antipathy from mother was modest at 0.23, p < 0.025 with 67% of pairs in agreement. The figures for father were higher at 0.42, p < 0.001 and 88% agreement in pairs.

14 Corroboration in sisters for antipathy from mother was 0.41, p < 0.001
    and 75% agreement in pairs. For father the figures were 0.50, p <
    0.0001 and 89% agreement in pairs.

Part II

Abuse

While the previous three chapters described neglectful parenting, the next three outline different types of abuse uncovered in our investigation of childhood, largely but not exclusively from parents. The three types of abuse – physical, sexual and psychological – proved to be related to neglect but all had features which made them distinct from experiences covered so far, and from each other. Unlike neglect, characteristics of abuse such as its frequency, the age when abuse started, relationship to perpetrator, and confiding about abuse were all more pertinent. In terms of the relationship to perpetrator, a wider sweep of individuals was covered. Parents and replacement parents were of greatest significance, but other household members were also included, and in the case of sexual abuse, perpetrators from wider kin or other parts of the community were included. Clearly multiple abuses were possible, from different perpetrators and in different family structures. Thus separate measurement of each abuse by each perpetrator was made. The prevalences of the abuses in the Representative series are covered, as well as examination of characteristics of the abuse and its severity in relation to adult depression.

As with neglect, the possible effects of abuse on childhood self-esteem, coping and relationships with others are examined. In addition, conduct problems such as frequent truanting, running away from home, aggression and rule-breaking are also considered. These were rare among the women we studied and largely unrelated to neglect but we found them to be more common in relation to abuse. In the case of psychological abuse we also extended the analysis to include alcohol or drug abuse and self-harm since preliminary analyses showed that depression was probably not the major consequence of this childhood experience.

Psychological abuse has only recently been identified by our own and other research teams, and thus we present only preliminary analyses. It proved to be very rare in our community series, which makes an extensive analysis difficult. However, we felt it merited inclusion in a discussion of abuse. We present definitions and descriptions of such abuse in the hope that this information can be utilised by other researchers and practitioners in contact with higher risk populations for such abuse in secure units, prisons and psychiatric hospitals.

Chapter 5

Physical abuse: beyond reasonable chastisement

> That societies to protect animals from cruelty were established before societies to protect children is one of the better known bizarre features of English social history. . . . Less well known perhaps, is that Parliament itself intervened to protect animals from abuse more than three-quarters of a century before it thought it proper to extend statutory protection to the young child. As in the case of infant life protection, so here, reluctance to legislate was rooted in the contemporary view that it was improper and, indeed, unsafe to invade the privacy of the home.
>
> (Pinchbeck and Hewitt 1973: 621–623)[1]

The public perception of the child as in need of protection from physical harm has historically been slow in evolving. Up until 1780 for example, the penal system permitted children to be hanged for minor offences. One tragic illustration of this is the case of a seven-year-old girl who was hanged for stealing a petticoat.[2] The harshness of the judicial system was mirrored by a greater concern for property than persons. Thus until the early nineteenth century it was not an offence in English law to steal a child unless it was clothed, and then the penalty reflected the value of the clothes. Mistreatment of family members by the male head of the household was considered almost a right in some quarters, and a matter beyond legislation. 'Wife beating and child-starving are facts that cannot be interfered with' declared an article appearing in the *Saturday Review* of 1857.[3] Since an Englishman's home was perceived to be his castle, the regulation of behaviour in the home remained the sole preserve of the male head of the household.

Although child protection has greatly improved this century, events still come to light which suggest that as a society progress is still faltering. In 1996 newspapers reported the case of a stepfather who was tried for 'assault occasioning actual bodily harm' following a severe thrashing he gave his nine-year-old son.[4] Medical evidence showed that the child had a series of weals inflicted across his legs and bottom over a period of a week. The jury ruled that the stepfather's actions fell within the realms of 'reasonable chastisement' of a child by a parent, and he was acquitted. 'Reasonable chastisement' represents a level of physical punishment which is permissible under English law. The child involved has since appealed against the decision and has taken his case to the European Court of Human Rights, where at the time of writing he is awaiting the final ruling on the matter. The outcome has significant implications for the rights of parents to use physical punishment against their children.

PUNISHMENT VERSUS ABUSE

Some would argue that the type of physical punishment described above, when carried out as a means of disciplining the child rather than as an assault *per se*, is not only necessary but commendable. Few would disagree that children must acquire a code of conduct to regulate behaviour, and that sanctions need to be imposed at times when behavioural boundaries are transgressed. The controversy arises in the use of *physical* chastisement as a means of regulating a child's behaviour. Even if physical chastisement is accepted in principle, the questions needing to be addressed concern what degree of physical discipline is appropriate and by what age is it appropriate to use it. An American survey on violence in the home reported that as many as 73 per cent of parents of two-year-olds have pushed, grabbed, shoved, slapped or smacked their child in the prior twelve months.[5] While these figures give no indication of how hard or frequently the children are slapped, doubtless a number of parents find themselves crossing the line between fair discipline and physical abuse. When the 'acceptable' level of physical discipline is exceeded, the short-term effects upon a child are usually evident – distress and upset, accompanied by physical injury. In the long term the effects are less visible, and may involve psychological damage. The aim of our research was to define the degree of physical harm which was capable of inflicting such long-term psychological damage.

An essential task in this process was to establish a threshold for what constituted physical abuse. This posed something of a challenge given the variation in social opinion on the topic. The threshold we chose for categorising an assault as abuse had to be set fairly high, given that we were searching for a type of maltreatment in childhood which might increase a woman's risk of depression as much as twenty years later. Some cases clearly reached such a threshold, where for example, a child was thrown downstairs, ferociously beaten or maimed for life. Other cases were less easy to categorise. Light 'smacks' on the hand or back of the leg, for example, were exceedingly common in the childhood histories we collected, and their inclusion would have led to the majority of women being classified as abused. We therefore set our threshold for abuse at a more severe level.

DEFINING PHYSICAL ABUSE

Our approach to defining abuse involved applying a standard set of criteria to case history material in order to arrive at a decision on the degree to which abuse had taken place. The system of categorisation had been developed beyond a simple dichotomy for classifying experiences as abusive or not, and allowed for descriptions of physical attacks to be graded for severity in much the same way as other forms of maltreatment described in previous chapters. This enabled us to investigate the relationship between different levels of abuse and adult outcomes.

In establishing the criteria used for grading severity of physical assaults, we first considered the characteristics of the violence itself: the degree of force used, how the child was hit, how often, and which part of the child's body was involved. However, the unpleasantness of the circumstances in which the attack was carried out was also considered relevant. The ferocity of the attack and the fury of the attacker contributed to a more severe rating. For example one woman said of her father: 'You could really gauge my father because his expression would change – his eyes would become quite manic. He definitely lost control without a doubt. You could see it happen. He would be sitting there and he would be annoyed. Then there would be an explosion and he was completely different. It would be very frightening.'

The unpredictable nature of attacks was also considered important, as in this example: 'I was doing the hoovering one day. A bit of dog biscuit rattled in it and mum was like a banshee coming through the kitchen screaming because she thought I was going to break the hoover. One minute I'm doing the hoovering and the next minute there's all these slaps around the back of my head. You never knew what you would do to set her off. The noise she made was frightening – the shouting and screaming – she did seem out of control.'

Other situations which increased the severity of the physical attacks were those involving public humiliation of the child. For example, when one woman's father discovered that she had been caught smoking at school and was caned by her teacher, she was punished again. In front of her mother, grandparents, aunt and uncle, her father put her over his knee, pulled down her knickers and belted her across her bare bottom. She was thirteen at the time. Her enduring memory of the incident is not so much the pain that the belt inflicted, but rather the humiliation of the public nature of the beating.

In addition to considering the features of the violence and the context in which it occurred, injuries sustained were also taken into account when ascertaining severity of abuse. The child's age and size were considered important given the differential impact a blow might have. A four-year-old might be thrown across the room by the force of a hard slap across the face, while the same attack on a fifteen-year-old might only result in a stinging, red cheek. Although injuries sustained by the child were of relevance, this was usually only insofar as it confirmed the severity of the attack. Given individual differences in capacity to bruise, we were reluctant to define abuse solely in terms of physical injury to the child. Some women survived appalling assaults as children with relatively superficial marks to show for what they had endured, and these attacks were nonetheless counted as abuse.

All the above aspects of assaults were taken into account in arriving at a definition of physical abuse. By careful summation of these factors we were able to grade women's experiences of childhood physical abuse, ranging from 'marked' through to 'moderate' and 'mild' levels of severity. The examples below are typical of the ratings we made under each level of severity.

'Marked' severity

The following is an example of a 'marked' attack administered by a child's father: 'From a very young age I was beaten around my face and head with a stick, or the heel of a shoe or a belt. It happened at least once a week. On one occasion when my dad hit me with his shoe, my tooth was knocked out. He beat me and beat me and beat me, and a neighbour had to pull him off me.' The violence in this example was frequent and involved the use of implements used as weapons, which were directed mostly at the head. The attack was clearly carried out with considerable force and in an uncontrolled manner. For this reason it was rated on the highest point of the severity scale.

'Moderate' severity

A typical example of a 'moderate' rating on the severity of abuse scale was the following: 'I was regularly caned on the lower half of the body from an early age. At other times mother would lose her temper, sometimes frighteningly, and give me a clip round the ear for answering her back. There were never any serious injuries as a result, I was just red and stinging for a while afterwards.' Although this abuse involved the use of an implement, the degree of force used and frequency of the assaults were less intense than those in the previous example.

'Mild' severity

Contrast the above examples with the following description of abuse received from a father: 'He would hit me hard with his hand or a rolled up newspaper but never around my face or head.' The latter was rated 'mild' in terms of severity, since it was infrequent and involved considerably less force than the other two examples. Mild abuse typically consisted of occasional single slaps across the face, or being hit on the legs with a slipper. In our analysis examining the relationship between abuse and depression we tested the threshold for what constituted physical abuse and showed that those rated 'mild' were unrelated to later disorder. Thus the following discussion of prevalence rates and perpetrators only includes those rated 'marked' or 'moderate'.

PREVALENCE OF PHYSICAL ABUSE

In our Representative London Women series 18 per cent of women reported physical abuse at 'marked' or 'moderate' levels during their childhoods.[6] This is similar to rates of neglect discussed in earlier chapters. Establishing an accurate prevalence rate for a sensitive topic such as physical abuse of children is a difficult task and raises much controversy. Estimates are criticised for under- or over-reporting the phenomenon depending on the means by which figures are collated. With respect to the prevalence rate reported here, we believe that if error is present then an under-estimate rather than over-estimate is the more likely.

One factor contributing to a possible under-estimate of the prevalence which we had to consider was that physical abuse may have occurred at a very young age and simply remained beyond recall. Figures from the NSPCC show that in 1975 the average age of the physically abused children on their 'risk' registers was three years and eight months, a figure similar to that found in the US.[7] By 1990 this figure had increased to age seven years and one month. Despite the increase in age, the figures demonstrate that reported physical abuse of children most commonly happens when very young, sometimes too young for a child to have a memory of it in adulthood. This is borne out by our research. Of the women who experienced physical abuse in our sample of sisters, the majority (75 per cent) experienced it before the age of ten, with 41 per cent of all severe physical abuse reported as beginning before the age of five.

Occasionally women were able to recount early instances of physical abuse because they had been told about it by an older family member, relative or neighbour. One woman's neighbour witnessed her physical abuse over the garden fence. The girl's father would hold her face and twist it hard if she cried as she lay in her pram. Many of the reports to the NSPCC rely on precisely such observations by relatives, neighbours and doctors. What remains uncertain is how much physical abuse lies undetected because it is conducted behind closed doors and the children themselves are too young to speak out.

PERPETRATORS OF PHYSICAL ABUSE

In our definition of physical abuse we only included attacks carried out by household members. By routinely asking about household abuse we were able to compare levels of abuse from mothers and fathers, surrogate parents, other caregivers and older siblings. This enabled us to examine not only who the most likely perpetrators were, but also who inflicted the most severe abuse. In the Representative

London Women sample, over half of the instances of 'marked' or 'moderate' abuses (56 per cent) were carried out by fathers or replacement fathers, compared with 23 per cent by mothers or surrogate mothers. A further 17 per cent of women experienced physical abuse at these levels from *both* mother and father. A small proportion (4 per cent) were abused by other household members, such as grandparents or brothers.[8]

Although fairly rare in the series, attacks from older brothers were often very severe, as this next example illustrates: 'My brother who was about ten years older than me used to take on the father role. If I came home with the wrong comic he'd asked me to bring back, it would be – bang! There'd be a smash across the face. I do remember a period where I was hit every night, whether I'd warranted it or not. When I was twelve he did hit me an awful lot, I mean he hit me so hard I had bruises on my arms and my eyes were black. He'd accused me of putting make-up on and I hadn't, and it ended up with about two hours of him hitting me and I was totally hysterical. My mother came in and saw what was happening and stood there shouting at me as well.' Such assaults from siblings or other household members are often overlooked in studies of physical abuse despite these attacks having the same potential for physical and psychological damage as those committed by parents.

In the Sisters series, the perpetrator of the abuse was just as likely to be a mother as a father. This may be a reflection of the selection procedure used in the Sisters study, whereby participants were selected largely for having difficult relationships with their mothers. However, it may also reflect our increasing thoroughness in more recent projects in routinely questioning about abuse from *each* parent figure instead of focusing on the worst instance. Other research in this area reports contradictory findings concerning the prevalence of abuse from mothers as opposed to fathers. One possible explanation for this inconsistent result concerns the inclusion threshold for severity of attacks and whether severity relates to the gender of perpetrator. When severity of abuse was examined in the Sisters series it was clear that fathers were responsible for the most serious attacks. As many as 22 per cent of assaults carried out by fathers were rated as 'marked' in severity, compared with 11 per cent carried out by mothers.[9] Thus studies which only categorise the parent responsible for the *most* severe attacks may emphasise the fathers' role and overlook lesser abuse by mothers.

THE CONTEXT OF PHYSICAL ABUSE

We used our Representative London Women series to examine the family structure in which physical abuse occurred. We found that physical abuse was most likely to occur in the context of a home headed by a natural parent and step-parent. Twice as many women (30 per cent) suffered instances of childhood physical abuse in such households compared to women who grew up in households headed by both natural parents (14 per cent).[10] Rates of physical abuse were *lowest* (8 per cent) in households headed by a single parent, most often a mother.

Physical abuse was also highly related to neglect in childhood. Half of the women who experienced parental neglect also suffered physical abuse compared with 10 per cent of those without neglect.[11] Physical abuse was also related to parental antipathy. Around a third of those with antipathy from mother suffered physical abuse compared with 15 per cent of those without antipathy.[12] The same figures applied to antipathy from father. A similar relationship held for family discord, with a third of such families physically abusing the child compared with 12 per cent of non-discordant families.

CHILDHOOD COPING WITH PHYSICAL ABUSE

In order to survive these brutal childhood experiences, children learnt to adapt as best they could. They often struggled to restore feelings of control and to regain their sense of self-worth by developing a number of physical and emotional strategies to cope with the abuse. Some women described spirited attempts to avoid punishment. One recounted how she managed to stay out of her father's vicious reach with great agility: 'He would hit me on the head and I would go flying. But I worked out some very good avoidance tactics. One was locking myself in the bathroom, the other was getting under the bed. If he tried to reach under the bed and hit me I would slide on the linoleum to the other side of the floor under the bed. When he ran round that side to hit me, I'd slide back again!'

Running away from home was another strategy some children employed to overcome the abuse. One woman recounted how she repeatedly absconded to escape her father's beatings, only to be brought back to the house by the police a day or two later. 'I can remember one incident where I ran into the lounge. The doors had locks, so I locked myself in, and he actually broke the door down. Being so frightened inside the room and seeing the splinters of wood, I opened the window and ran away, and he was chasing me. I'd probably been exceptionally naughty, I don't know, but I knew it was going to be a big wallop if he found me.' Some children managed to escape without detection by the police, and never returned home again. Not surprisingly, many runaways are the products of abusive households such as these. A recent study of homeless youth in London (using the same measures of physical abuse) found that over half had been severely physically abused in childhood.[13] Other youngsters in our samples left home as soon as they were able to support themselves financially, and in a quarter of instances of abuse this was the reason for the abuse ending.

In addition to running away, another method of coping with the abuse was retaliation in the form of threats. This tactic was usually adopted in teenage years, when the girls were physically stronger and felt able to challenge the abuser. A common experience was the following: 'Once my mother gave me a black eye when I was about fifteen, and I told her: "If you ever hit me again, I'm telling you – mother or no mother – I'll hit you back."' Few teenagers actually did hit back. In most cases the threats they made were sufficient to reduce or even terminate the abuse. Standing up to the abuser in this way often restored the child's sense of self-worth and autonomy, as one woman recounted: 'I remember making a stand against my older sister when I was about ten and saying to her "No, you're not always going to tell me what to do", and I remember the feeling then of becoming my own person, not under her power. She stopped hitting me after that.' In one in ten instances the abuse was terminated by the child's assertive actions as in the above example.

Sometimes the girls became not only assertive but aggressive: 'My stepfather gave me a black eye once, so I kicked him back. He also hit me on the face – I ran up to my room and trapped his hand in the door. I answered him back and swore at him. I kicked him in the balls!' At times such violent retaliation led to even worse beatings for the child, as one girl discovered: 'I got a really good hiding for slapping my mother. When my stepfather came home he punched me across the top of the head which sent me hurtling backwards. I suddenly snapped and the next thing the two of us were on the passage floor fighting like two men. I scratched him very severely down his cheek and throat until I saw blood. And all I could think of was, ''I'm going to hurt you as much as you hurt me.'' ' When we looked at conduct problems in childhood and teenage years involving aggression and rule-breaking behaviour, these were three times as common among women who had suffered physical abuse. Some 13 per cent of women with abuse reported at least three such conduct problems compared with 4 per cent of other women.[14]

In contrast to these defiant responses, other women reported that they were rendered helpless by the physical abuse, immobilised by feelings of constant fear.[15] This was particularly true when the attacks were unpredictable. One girl's father maintained a reign of terror in the household by means of random, brutal assaults on all the family: 'When dad came home from the pub he'd get mum by the head, and he would bash her head off the white enamel sink, and we were all screaming as we watched.' His anger could be triggered by the slightest thing: 'He threw his dinner on the floor when he didn't like it. He was drunk and he just chucked it off the table and the plate broke and split my toe.' On another occasion: 'He beat us with the strap of a suitcase once because we asked to go to the park on a Sunday afternoon. Even though the other children's parents were offering to take us, he wouldn't let us go. He beat us instead.' Other women told of similar aggressive outbursts prompted by the most insignificant comment or action on the part of the child: 'The attack was out of the blue. Dad was peeling potatoes with my mum and he wasn't that keen on doing it and I came in and said to him you've missed a bit and he just went for me with the knife at my throat.'

As a means of survival in such relentlessly abusive conditions, some children acquired the skill of attuning to the mood of the abuser and placating him or her when the antecedents of an assault seemed on the horizon. In these households children lived on tenterhooks, awaiting any signal that warned of the next attack. This 'frozen watchfulness', as it has been called, is a perpetual state of tense vigilance resulting from frequent but random assaults.[16] One woman describes the constant state of terror that both she, her sisters and their mother experienced as a result of her father's random, unprovoked violence: 'You felt tense when he was there and tense when he wasn't, because you were thinking, is he going to come in any minute now.' She tried to anticipate and diffuse any situation that might trigger her drunken father's ferocious temper: 'I used to run around to try to humour him so that he wouldn't cause a row or wreck the place. But it's left me with a fear of drunks – I don't even like my husband to have a drink.'

Some children made desperate attempts to appease the abuser. Women described how they displayed the utmost obedience in the vain hope of deterring an attack. Many rationalised the violence by telling themselves that they must be to blame for the beatings they received, and that if only they were to become a 'good girl' the violence might stop. As with the neglectful experiences described in earlier chapters, children who were physically abused felt highly stigmatised and ashamed. Many became isolated and lonely and exhibited a high degree of helplessness in childhood. These experiences were not specific to physical abuse: they appeared to accompany several forms of childhood mistreatment.[17]

PHYSICAL ABUSE AND ADULT DEPRESSION

In the Representative London Women series, 33 per cent of women with physical abuse in childhood were depressed in the year of study compared with 14 per cent of non-abused women.[18] Similar results held in the Sisters series. When the relationship between severity of abuse and rates of adult psychiatric disorder in our samples were examined, a finding emerged which highlighted the significance of grading experiences of abuse. Rates of depression among those who had experienced 'mild' abuse were very similar to those for women who had experienced no physical abuse in childhood (19 per cent and 17 per cent respectively). By comparison, 33 per cent of those who experienced 'moderate' abuse and 41 per cent of those who suffered 'marked' abuse were depressed in the year of interview.[19] The latter finding hints at the reason why estimates of the prevalence of abuse vary from study to study. The inclusion of very minor instances of abuse results on the one hand in artificially high prevalence rates and on the other hand in a dilution of the relationship between physical abuse and adult depression. Thus, the criteria one sets for defining abuse are central to any investigation of abuse.

THE SECRETIVENESS OF PHYSICAL ABUSE

We did not discount or down-rate the severity of an attack if there was an absence of medical treatment or official intervention. In the scores of abuse histories collected, only a handful of women received medical treatment for their injuries and even fewer reached the attention of agencies such as social services or the NSPCC. In the Sisters series for example, only one in ten women with severe physical abuse received any official contact or intervention.[20] Women learnt to lie about the abuse from an early age in order to cover it up. 'We knew what to say – "I walked into the door" or "I tripped". We were told not to tell.' On the whole, abusing parents avoided official contacts, maintaining a low profile for fear of detection. Fear was also the overriding reason why the children were actively discouraged from seeking help. Worse reprisals were threatened if such disclosure ever took place.[21] The terror instilled in the child by threats of further severe beatings was a powerful deterrent to disclosure of the abuse to the outside world. Indeed, only 17 per cent of women severely abused in the Sisters series actually confided in someone about the attacks at the time.[22]

Fear was the reason for one girl not pursuing the case against her father with social services: 'When I was fourteen or fifteen, I actually ran away from home. I told one of my friends about the abuse, who then told one of the teachers. She took me to one side and then went to my head of year and then the social services. I suppose I felt brave and thought "Yes, they can do something about it", until I went to social services and they said "It's not as easy as the teacher made it out to be. You'll have to go home until we can sort something out for you." I thought "I'm not going to be exposed to that." If he knows that I've been there, then that's it. I might as well start digging my grave now. I dropped all the charges against him.'

Sometimes the injuries from the abuse were noticed at school. One woman's drunken stepfather used to return from the pub, 'to punch me, pull my hair, and throw me down the stairs, or belt me until he took the skin off my back'. The social services were alerted to the maltreatment after an observant teacher noticed her bruises and cuts. Her parents colluded in describing the home as a happy one, and explained away her injuries as minor accidents. Social services took their enquiries no further, as they were fully convinced by the parent's persuasive lies. Following this incident her stepfather began to apply more psychological methods of abuse which left no visible marks. These are described in a later chapter.

The above examples show how instances of support from adults outside the family were at times thwarted by the cleverness of the abuser. However, sometimes the support was effective. One woman received support from a close adult friend who persuaded her to make a stand against her abusing father, much to his annoyance: 'I'd been banned from seeing her because he said she was a bad influence on me, that was really hard. We'd suddenly become like sisters, somebody older than me that I could turn to.' At age fifteen she confronted her father, after accepting his punishments for five years. 'He never struck me after that. I realised she had been right, I had to stand my ground.'

MINIMISING THE REPORTING OF ABUSE

Instances of physical abuse were generally recalled quite readily by the women we interviewed. However, to a greater extent than with neglect, accounts of physical abuse were reported in a low-key way, with women attempting to 'normalise' the experience.[23] For example, after describing an assault by her father one woman said: 'There was no violence, no *intended* violence. He wasn't bothered, we weren't bothered – it wasn't enough to get your emotions going, it was just a belt.' Another woman's account of her father's violence seemed quite innocuous at first, but the severity gradually became apparent: 'I was beaten, but I was never really physically harmed that I needed to cover myself up to go to school. I was just hit around the head or kicked or shoved out of the way, or stuck in the coal cellar. He tried to strangle me once.'

Many expressions were used to minimise the violence of the attack. These included being 'clipped around the ear' or 'having your ears boxed'. What was described as a clip around the ear by one woman on further questioning turned out to be a severe beating around the head which resulted in a bleeding mouth. Some women viewed physical abuse as a 'normal' or typical part of their upbringing, particularly when used as punishment for bad behaviour. Their reluctance to distinguish physical punishment from physical abuse was reflected in comments such as: 'All the kids in our street got hit like that when they misbehaved.' Other women sought to vindicate their parents, stressing how deserving they were of chastisement, with comments such as 'I'd been very naughty, he'd warned me before.' Such justifications were not allowed to influence *our* assessment of the severity of the abuse. We attended to the characteristics of the violence itself rather than the woman's perception of how deserving she was of the attack or how normal the attack was in her experience.

THE EXPERIENCES OF SISTERS

Obtaining an accurate estimate of the prevalence of physical abuse is particularly difficult when there are few official records of the phenomenon. Since only a handful of the instances of abuse in our series ever came to the attention of official bodies, validating documentation simply did not exist for the bulk of the data. This is where accounts of abusive instances collected from independent observers of the scene are key, and for this reason the Sisters project was extremely valuable. Sisters were independently interviewed and asked not only about their own childhood experience but also about what they had observed happening to their sister. The account of childhood abuse that one sister said she experienced was compared to the account recalled by her sister. There was remarkable agreement between sisters on ratings of each other's physical abuse: 84 per cent of pairs agreed on the exact degree of abuse that the other had received.[24] One of the reasons that sisters were able to report so accurately on each other was that both commonly suffered the same degree of maltreatment and witnessed it happening to each other.[25] In three-quarters of instances sisters endured the same degree of abuse (76 per cent agreement).

CONCLUSION

As a result of a century of social and legislative change, the physical abuse of many more children has been acknowledged. It now seems extraordinary that earlier in the century doctors were actually considering as a new clinical disorder certain multiple fractures to infants. These puzzlingly cleared up when children were taken into hospital care, and spontaneously reappeared when they were returned to their home environment.[26] While the numbers of children placed on risk registers show no sign of a down-turn, these figures nevertheless are a testimony to the increasing willingness of society to acknowledge physical abuse, and to protect more children than ever before from its harmful effects.

While the detection of physical abuse remains paramount, the prevention of such abuse must also be a long-term goal. Legislation banning corporal punishment of children by parents already exists in five European countries (Sweden, Finland, Norway, Cyprus and Austria). However, parents also need assistance in learning to cope with the demands of child-rearing. Everyday stresses such as work or the strain of unemployment, financial hardship or marital problems doubtless contribute to a readiness by parents to take out their frustrations on their children. There are also parents who find themselves too emotionally handicapped by their own experience of childhood neglect or abuse to provide adequate care for their own children. Prevention of child abuse therefore holds promise not only for the children of today but also for future generations who will be the parents of tomorrow.

NOTES

1 Pinchbeck, I. and Hewitt, M. (1973) *Children in English Society*, vol. II, London: Routledge and Kegan Paul.
2 Ibid.
3 'Wife-beating', *Saturday Review*, 16 May 1857, vol. 3, no. 81: 446–447.
4 See for example: 'Parents could face new restrictions on smacking children', *Guardian* 10 September 1996.
5 Wauchope, B.A. and Strauss, M.A. (1990) 'Physical punishment and physical abuse of American children: incidence rates by age, gender, and occupational class', in Strauss, M.A. and Gelles, R.J. (eds) *Physical Violence in American Families – Risk Factors and Adaptations to Violence in 8145 Families*, New Brunswick, NJ: Transaction.
6 The prevalence of physical abuse in the Representative London Women series was 18% (52/286).
7 Creighton, S.J. (1992) *Child Abuse Trends in England and Wales 1988–1990*, London: NSPCC.
8 Among 52 women with 'marked' or 'moderate' abuse in the Representative series, 56% (29) had physical abuse solely from a father figure, 23% (12) solely from a mother figure and 17% (9) from both mother and father. A further 4% (2) had physical abuse from another household member.
9 In the Sisters series 79 women experienced physical abuse at 'marked' or 'moderate' levels of severity by at least one perpetrator. If multiple abuses are counted then there were 99 by different perpetrators. There were a further 35 instances of mild abuse. Of the 65 abuses by father figure 22% (14) were 'marked', 51% (33) 'moderate' and 28% (18) 'mild'. Of the 64 abuses by mother the figures were 11% (7), 64% (41) and 25% (16) respectively (5 further abuses were from other household members of which 2 were 'marked', 2 'moderate' and 1 'mild').
10 In the Representative London Women series, for all household arrangements in childhood (N = 465, 1.6 per person) the highest rate of physical abuse was in families headed by a parent and step-parent where the rate was 30% (8/27). The rate of physical abuse with both natural parents was 14% (39/282) and for families headed by a lone parent the rate was 8% (5/65) with other arrangements having a rate of 9% (8/91) of physical abuse (p < 0.05).

11 *Table 5.1* Physical abuse and neglect (Representative London Women series)

Neglect	% physical abuse
Present	56 (28/50)
Absent	10 (24/236)
	$p < 0.001$

12 *Table 5.2* Physical abuse, antipathy and discord (Representative London Women series) (% physical abuse)

Experience	Antipathy from mother	Antipathy from father	Family discord
Present	34 (17/50)	36 (20/56)	36 (27/75)
Absent	15 (35/236)	14 (32/230)	12 (28/211)
	$p < 0.001$	$p < 0.001$	$p < 0.001$

13 Craig, T., Hodson, S., Woodward, S. and Richardson, S. (1996) *Off to a Bad Start*, London: Mental Health Foundation Report, 19 November, UMDS, St Thomas's Hospital, London.

14 *Table 5.3* Physical abuse and three or more conduct problems in childhood (Sisters series)

Physical abuse	% with conduct problems
Present	13 (10/79)
Absent	4 (5/119)
	$p < 0.10$

15 *Table 5.4* Physical abuse and childhood helplessness (Sisters series)

Physical abuse	% helpless
Present	27 (21/79)
Absent	12 (14/119)
	$p < 0.025$

16 Herman, J. (1992) *Trauma and Recovery*, London: Pandora; USA: Basic Books.

17   *Table 5.5* Physical abuse and relations to others (Sisters series)

Physical abuse	% felt shame	% loneliness
Present	59 (47/79)	49 (39/79)
Absent	33 (39/119)	31 (37/119)
	p < 0.001	p < 0.05

18   *Table 5.6* Physical abuse and adult depression (% depressed)

Physical abuse	Representative London Women series	Sisters series
Present	33 (17/52)	35 (28/79)
Absent	14 (33/234)	18 (21/119)
	p < 0.005	p < 0.01

19   *Table 5.7* Severity of peak worst physical abuse and depression (Sisters series)

Severity	% depressed
a. Marked	41 (9/22)
b. Moderate	33 (19/57)
c. Mild	19 (4/21)
d. None	17 (17/98)

a and b vs c and d   p < 0.01

20 In the Sisters series, for those 99 instances of 'marked' or 'moderate' physical abuse, official contact (with police, social or educational services) held for 10%. Official intervention was responsible for only 3% of abuses ending.
21 Secretiveness was imposed by perpetrator in 10% of such abuse instances in the Sisters series.
22 Some 17% of abuse incidents were disclosed to others and 14% received a supportive response.
23 Reluctance to report the physical abuse at interview held for 14% of instances of abuse in the Sisters series.
24 Corroboration in sister pairs was 0.57 (p < 0.001) with 84% of pairs in agreement over the degree of physical abuse.
25 Concordance in the sister pairs was 0.40 (p < 0.0001) with 76% of pairs having similar experience of physical abuse.
26 Gilham, B. (1994) *The Facts about Child Physical Abuse*, London, New York: Cassell.

Chapter 6

Sexual abuse: shared secrecy and guilt

> Lolita! Light of my life, fire of my loins. My sin, my soul! . . .
> Overtly I had so-called normal relationships with a number of
> terrestrial women . . . inly I was consumed by a hell furnace of
> localised lust for every passing nymphet. I would tell myself that
> it was all a question of attitude, that there was really nothing
> wrong in being moved to distraction by girl-children . . . those
> over eight but under fourteen years of age.
>
> (Nabokov 1959: 9)[1]

The sexual abuse of children is not a new phenomenon. Documentation throughout this century attests to its common occurrence. It is
known, for example, that even in Victorian England there were tens
of thousands of child prostitutes and Freud encountered descriptions
of incest among his first patients seen prior to the First World War.
Sexual abuse was also documented in Kinsey's report of sexual
behaviour in the US in the late 1940s. It has also been a fairly
frequent theme in literature: the explicit description of abuse of a
thirteen-year-old in Nabokov's *Lolita* appeared in the late 1950s.
And yet sexual abuse has only become a major focus of attention by
researchers and health professionals since the 1980s. Its long delay
in coming to public recognition has led to a fervour about its
identification, to the extent that it now appears to be the most
targeted childhood abusive experience. Reasons for its late recognition as a prevalent form of abuse are complex. One reason is that it
is still probably the most secret and covert of all the abuses. It is also
the most stigmatising, for both the perpetrator and the victim. This
inhibits disclosure and help-seeking on the part of the abused child.
The usual abhorrence most adults feel about childhood sexual abuse
may also account for some of the past dismissiveness of its likely

prevalence. Sexual abuse has also always aroused controversy, especially where verification of its occurrence is concerned. On the one hand in the 1980s there was an outcry that the founder of psychoanalysis dismissed reports of sexual abuse as fantasy.[2] On the other hand there was outrage at what was perceived as the mis-identification of sexual abuse on the basis of medical evidence, as in the Cleveland case in 1988.[3] A recent controversy gripping the public imagination involving sexual abuse concerns 'false memory syndrome'. This controversy has focused on litigation in the US where defendants have claimed to recover memories of abuse while undergoing psychotherapy and have brought proceedings, typically against their fathers, in adult life. A heated debate has ensued about whether these abuses actually occurred and were only re-remembered in adult life, or were solely the product of suggestion by over-zealous psychotherapists. The debate simultaneously revolves around whether childhood amnesia for early sexual abuse means that victims are unable to recall it except under psychotherapeutic intervention.[4]

The issue of whether people can accurately remember childhood experiences of sexual abuse is clearly crucial for the research we had undertaken. The long passage of time between the childhood experience and its recollection at interview means there was a possibility of the woman forgetting or distorting what occurred. We felt that this was no more likely to be true of sexual abuse than any other negative experience in childhood. We hoped that our analysis of pairs of sisters would give us some idea of whether the extent of corroboration for sexual abuse was similar to other mal-treatment.

Assessing abuse on the basis of adults' early memories has certain advantages over studying very recent abuse in children. Since the abuses ended some years ago, the ethical issues over intervening to halt the abuse were no longer pertinent. Another advantage is that since most of the women were no longer in contact with the abuser and none were engaged in litigation against an abuser, they clearly had nothing to gain from fabricating any account of abuse. We saw no reason why we could not ask about sexual abuse in a similar manner to asking about any other childhood experiences covered in our interviews.

' However, this is not to say that questioning about sexual abuse during interviews was easy. Most adults find the notion of children being used for sexual purposes distasteful and shocking. It is thus difficult both for women to talk about their experiences and for interviewers to ask questions with ease. Sometimes a woman's hesitancy in recounting her abuse revolved around the naming of body parts and describing sexual acts. Sometimes the descriptions were hesitant and disjointed, reflecting a woman's reconstruction of experience that she had probably not fully understood at the time of the abuse. Emotions surrounding sexual abuse are also complex. Often the abuse occurred in what appeared to be an affectionate context, the enjoyment of which caused feelings of guilt. Alternatively the victim may have been blamed for bringing it about, engendering feelings of self-reproach.

DEFINING SEXUAL ABUSE

One of the major problems of both identifying and studying childhood sexual abuse is that there has been little uniformity in its definition in terms of the degree of sexual contact and its frequency, or the relationship with the perpetrator. Thus some approaches have restricted the study of abuse to contact occurring between fathers and daughters, others include abuse from any kin while yet others have encompassed abuse from any perpetrator. Similarly, some studies have restricted their definition of an abusive situation to that between child and adult only, ignoring rapes by boyfriends and peers. Others have only included abuses where full sexual intercourse occurred, regardless of its frequency, while others have considered repeated abuse only as of significance, whether or not involving sexual intercourse.[5]

Of course all of these are potentially relevant and require investigation. In our own approach we adopted as broad a definition of sexual abuse as possible in order to test which experiences were most related to adult disorder. It was not always obvious to us what would cause greatest long-term harm. Although sexual intercourse with a father was clearly one of the most severe forms of childhood abuse, we felt that a rape by a stranger was also potentially damaging, as was repeated sexual exploitation by a person in authority such as a teacher or priest. We therefore decided to include examples of sexual abuse committed by any perpetrator in a range of contexts. Although most instances involved physical contact, we allowed some non-contact experiences to be included where the child was forced to witness sexual activity or look at, or be used for, pornographic material. We decided, however, to exclude the most common non-contact experiences such as seeing an exhibitionist, except when it was a relative or someone known to the child.

The type of mistreatment of children covered in previous chapters has involved distortions of parenting surrounding failures of care, control and responsibility for young children. In our definition of sexual abuse, however, exploitation of a child for sexual gratification by *any* adult is included, not sexual exploitation exclusively by parents. It thus takes in a wider social context, since we found that the *majority* of perpetrators were *not* natural parents. Sexual abuse therefore had to take into account other individuals the child came into contact with such as other relatives, family friends, school contacts and neighbours. But in common with the other types of neglect and abuse, the abuser plays on the child's powerlessness, violates the child's human rights and, given that most abusers are known to the child, betrays trust. Since it is an experience found stigmatising and shocking to most people it is difficult to disclose. As with adult rape some element of stigma inexplicably attaches to the victim and it is common for the victim to feel guilty and blameworthy for the sexual contact.

We set ourselves the task of assessing the severity of the abuses, taking all the potentially damaging and unpleasant aspects into account. Gradings of abuse were made in exactly the same way as for other childhood experiences already outlined. We took the two highest points of 'marked' or 'moderate' as denoting a serious or severe form of abuse. Those rated 'mild' were also analysed but were expected to result in less long-term psychological damage. In order to judge severity we routinely took into account the degree of sexual contact (in particular involving any form of penetration); the frequency of abuse, the age when it began, and the relationship to the perpetrator. We also took into account any particularly frightening or additionally unpleasant features such as enforced secrecy maintained by threats to others.

'Marked' severity

Most instances of sexual intercourse and most abuse by fathers, stepfathers and brothers were rated 'marked' on severity. Violent attacks, or those of greater frequency were also rated in this category. The following example is of sexual abuse by a stepfather which occurred when the child returned home after institutional care. Although initially it involved touching of her genitals it developed into regular sexual intercourse. 'He interfered with me. It started when I was seven and went on until I was eleven. It happened once a week or more. I couldn't tell anyone. I was such a young child. You're petrified of this man in the house, you're told not to tell. But my mother caught him herself and that was the end of that. I was put back in the orphanage. That's why she sent me away. She found out.'

Examples were usually considered severe when they were repeated experiences of sexual intercourse by close family members, but abuse by figures in authority also qualified, even when intercourse itself did not occur. In the following example the abuse is considered 'marked' on severity because it was repeated, the perpetrator was an authority figure, and because he threatened to kill the child's mother if she told anyone: 'I was abused by a schoolteacher for several months when I was eight. He took me to his house, saying he was going to show me his butterflies. He wasn't showing me his butterflies. He took me up to his bedroom. He'd try and keep me behind after school. It happened twice at his home and a few instances after school. Other girls knew – they used to tease me. I had to stroke him, play with him. He made me play with his willy in the cloakrooms. He used to try and rub himself on me and then he'd put all his sperm on my body – it was horrible. He used to say if I told anyone my mum was going to die. At the time I told no one at all. He left the school in the end because he used to try and touch other girls as well.'

'Moderate' severity

Examples in the 'moderately' severe category commonly involved repeated abuse from an unrelated adult but not involving sexual intercourse, or alternatively abuse on one occasion only from a trusted person such as a relative, close family friend or authority figure. The following example demonstrates repeated instances of abuse by a grandfather: 'It was my dad's dad. I was about nine or ten when it happened. He used to say to me "Go and get the Sunday paper and bring it through to me." So I went and got it from the letter box and he said "Come into the bed with papa, give papa a kiss and I'll give you two shillings." Apparently he used to have lots of girls and he used to tell me about it. As I got older he'd come in and say, "Oh, I was with this girl tonight", and go on like this to me and it used to really upset me because of my gran. At thirteen, I remember he took out his thing [penis] one night and I was just petrified and I used to run away but I couldn't tell my grandmother because it would have upset her too much. He tried to get my hand to touch it but I wouldn't let him. I knew it was wrong. He exposed himself about five times when I was between thirteen and fifteen.'

Some of the abuses occurred at a very young age and this was taken into consideration when rating the severity. The following abuse occurred when the child was under five, a factor taken into account when arriving at the 'moderate' severity rating. 'It was when I was three or four and my mother's boyfriend made me masturbate him. I never told anyone as a child, only my very close friends know. I can remember as if I was still there. I was sitting on his legs. I can see the room, the bed, the carpet, the walls, everything. He made me put my hands around his penis and move my hands up and down. I don't know how long it lasted for, maybe a few minutes. It seemed like forever. Then I heard my mum shouting. And immediately I felt immense guilt. I thought "What am I doing?" I remember running into the kitchen and being told off for something I'd done, and relating that to what was happening. That made it difficult to make contact with my mother in any way, really.'

'Mild' severity

'Mild' severity of sexual abuse typically involved single incidents with strangers of more minor touching not involving penetration. We routinely collected such examples to see if the threshold of severity selected was the correct one in predicting long-term psychological damage. While 'mild' abuses were often distressing occurrences for the child at the time, we believed long-term damage was less likely. An example of a mild abuse was the following incident which occurred once only when the child was age seven and living in local authority care. The church deacon asked her to help him carry books back to the church. 'He stood me on a table and kept touching my leg and putting his hand under my dress, running his hand down my back and stroking my hair . . . inside my pants, doing things he shouldn't have been doing. He was only probing, he didn't actually put his finger inside, he was just touching. He didn't say anything, just "Shut up and stand there" kind of thing. I was afraid, there was nobody around. I felt very ashamed. I never mentioned it to anyone until I was sixteen. It was a one-off encounter.'

The following 'mild' abuse was by a friend of the family when the girl was eight. 'He had a wife and a young daughter. On Sundays our families used to go to the football club and have a drink. We used to sometimes go back to their home. He had a big shed in his garden. He told me and my sister that he'd got some lovely rabbits in the shed. When we went to look he got his penis out and we ran out of the shed. It felt like a very frightening thing to tell our parents about. We actually said to him, "We're not going to say anything."'

PREVALENCE OF SEXUAL ABUSE

Different studies have shown a wide range of prevalences of sexual abuse. This is likely to be the result of different sampling procedures, different age groups studied and different definitions of abuse. Thus rates as high as 54 per cent and as low as 7 per cent have been reported for women. Where contact abuse is concerned rates of around 11 per cent are quoted.[6] In our Representative sample, sexual abuse involving physical contact occurred for 9 per cent of women.[7] Thus, among this group of women sexual abuse was only half as common as neglect or physical abuse.

CHARACTERISTICS OF SEXUAL ABUSE

In the Sisters series, when characteristics of childhood sexual abuse were examined in more detail it was found that women often suffered more than one experience of sexual abuse. About a third of women in the Sisters series with sexual abuse had suffered abuse in childhood by more than one perpetrator. Many of the abuses were frequent, with over a third of severe abuses taking place at least monthly. In terms of intrusiveness of sexual contact, around a third involved sexual intercourse and nearly half involved penetration of vagina or anus. There was no relationship to age, with severe abuses occurring equally in the three age bands: five or under, aged 6–10, and aged 11–17.

Although as many as a third of sexual abuses in our Representative series of women were committed by father or surrogate father, the majority were from other perpetrators including relatives, acquaintances and strangers. A quarter of sexual abuses were by other kin members, a fifth by family friends or acquaintances, and a quarter by strangers. Nearly all the perpetrators were male. Comparable figures on perpetrators were reported both in the Sisters and Adult Risk series.

THE CONTEXT OF SEXUAL ABUSE

Analysis of family structure in the Representative London Women series showed that sexual abuse occurred most commonly in step-parent families. Sexual abuse took place in 11 per cent of such households, although the stepfathers themselves were not necessarily the perpetrators. The level of abuse was similarly high in 'other' care arrangements including institutional care, care by other kin members or unrelated people looking after the children (9 per cent). Sexual abuse was only half as common in families headed by both natural parents or lone parents, usually the mother (4 per cent).[8]

Sexual abuse was highly correlated with neglect. It appeared that neglect of a child tended to occur at an earlier age, leaving the child prey to adults, often non-household members, who saw the child as vulnerable and a suitable victim. Being identifiable as a victim may also be the reason for a high correlation between sexual abuse outside the home and physical abuse in the home. There was no relationship, however, between sexual abuse and antipathy from either mother or father.[9]

Sexual abuse has some distinctive characteristics when compared to parental neglect and physical abuse. First, nearly all the sexual abusers proved to be male, therefore sexual abuse to girls involves a very specific power relationship involving gender. By comparison the perpetrators of physical abuse and neglect involved both male and female perpetrators. The second distinctive feature of sexual abuse is that the perpetrator is very often an adult from outside the household. Thus sexual abuse perpetration involves a wider social, kin and neighbourhood arena than other abuses. Another unique feature of sexual abuse is its frequent incomprehensibility to the young child at the time it occurs as a result of the child's sexual ignorance and immaturity. It is possible that the difficult cognitive processing of memories of abuse has a more complex impact on the self than other traumatic experiences. Often women reported that while they found the incidents unpleasant when they occurred, their main impact did not hit them until years afterwards.

THE SECRETIVENESS OF SEXUAL ABUSE

In order to obtain the child's compliance and also to maintain secrecy, perpetrators applied subtle methods of control and domination. Such emotional or psychological abuse will be explored more fully in the next chapter, and is well illustrated in Nabokov's *Lolita* quoted at the beginning of this chapter. Having abused his thirteen-year-old stepdaughter following her mother's death, Humbert keeps her virtual prisoner and swears her to secrecy about the abuse. He threatens her with abandonment knowing she has no close family or friends to protect her: 'What happens if you complain to the police of my having kidnapped and raped you? Let us suppose they believe you . . . so I go to jail. But what happens to you, my orphan? Well you are luckier. You become the ward of the Department of Public Welfare – which I'm afraid sounds a little bleak. . . . I don't know if you have ever heard of the laws relating to dependent, neglected, incorrigible and delinquent children . . . you will be given a choice of dwelling places, all more or less the same, the correctional school, the reformatory, the juvenile detention home. In plainer words, if we two are found out you will be analyzed and institutionalised. . . . This is the situation, this is the choice. Don't you think that in the situation Dolores Haze had better stick to her old man? . . . I succeeded in terrorising Lo . . . I managed to establish the background of shared secrecy and shared guilt' (Nabokov 1959: 151, see note 1).

Most of the incidents of sexual abuse in our series of women were kept secret, especially the more severe ones where a third of the women were either threatened or bribed into secrecy.[10] In the Sisters series 83 per cent of the sexual abuses were never disclosed in childhood. Disclosure was more common, however, where the abuse was mild, presumably because there was less stigma attached and less conflict of loyalty since such close family members were less likely to be involved. Secretiveness was imposed by the abuser in nearly a quarter of cases, nearly always severe abuses. Children were often threatened with violence to their siblings or mother if they did not comply with the abusers' wishes. One woman's siblings were beaten if she did not comply with her father's sexual demands: 'I used to feel guilty because my sister and brothers were getting beaten, whereas half the time he would just leave me. They'd think, ''Oh, you didn't get hit, why?'''

Other abusers were more subtle and relied for compliance on the child's low self-esteem and isolation from potential support, as in this example of sexual abuse by a father: 'I felt power over him, which was stupid really, because I was letting him abuse me. It didn't make me feel special to my dad, maybe because it started so early, I didn't think about it. It wasn't a secret exactly, it just happened. The reason for the ending of the abuse was about me developing a greater sense of myself and I thought "What are you doing?" and I stopped speaking to him, I stopped having anything to do with him. I didn't speak with my dad for about a year. I think going to an all-girls secondary school was very important. I was gradually being a lot more comfortable and assertive and I think I'd say "no" and avoid situations where I'd be on my own with my dad. If he'd call me, I'd not go and I stopped speaking to him. I was keeping him at a distance. Once he said "Come here" and I thought "No way am I going to go there" and "I'll never have anything to do with you again". He'd really invaded me – he had no right to do that.'

In another instance a father built up his daughter's reputation as a liar so that if she did tell anyone she wouldn't be believed: 'He would make me out to be a liar. I think it was like preparing in case I ever did say anything.' Another girl was actually branded a liar for disclosing the abuse from her grandfather: 'It was more for a cry for help that I told my mum. Then when my dad confronted him and he denied it, I was accused of being a liar, it was awful. After that grandfather was saying that I was asking for it, that I was the one doing all the leading.'

Unfortunately the abuser often has the collusion of other people both in the family and in authority. In the past there has been a good deal of resistance to uncovering abuse. Some have criticised female partners of sexual abusers for failing to intervene to prevent or stop the abuse. We came across some instances of mothers who seemed helpless to intervene, lacked insight or simply seemed unable to confront the full horror of the situation. We can only guess at their reasons for non-intervention. One woman said: 'I told my mother about father running out of the room when he was disturbed abusing me. I don't remember her making the connection or saying anything to me. All I can remember is telling her and that was it, nothing more. On one occasion, mother said "You would tell me if your Dad was being 'familiar', wouldn't you?" and I didn't.' In another case a mother not only disbelieved that her boyfriend was abusing her thirteen-year-old daughter, but as a result of the daughter's disclosure actually moved the boyfriend into the house, allowing the abuse to increase.

The following example tells of a girl who tried to inform authorities that she was being sexually abused by her father: 'I told my school but wasn't believed. When I first told them my dad was abusing me they got a doctor in. She kept showing me these books with men and saying, ''Is this what your dad looks like, is this what he's doing?'' I just freaked out in the end. They just turned round and said I was attention-seeking. I wasn't believed until I was sixteen. My dad made me promise not to tell anyone. ''It's our secret'' he used to say.'

COPING WITH SEXUAL ABUSE IN CHILDHOOD

There were a variety of responses to sexual abuse among the women we interviewed. Some children were petrified. Others, although uncomfortable about the abuse, were not actually scared. A number described the dissociative 'out of the body experiences' commonly linked with sexual abuse. Many of the women developed much stronger feelings about the abuse later in life when they could consider it more objectively. They sometimes felt betrayed by mothers whom they described as failing to protect them. They also felt angry at the perpetrator. Many felt stigmatised and tainted for years after the experience.

'Disavowal' of the experience of abuse was fairly common, although women were still able to tell us the main details of what had occurred. For example one woman was able to give a description of her abuse, and yet said: 'I don't really remember and to be honest with you I don't want to remember. I blanked it out. It never happened.' Another said: 'I was terrified and I froze. If I have any dreams connected with it I'm numb from the waist down.' Or a similar response: 'At the time I thought, ''Get it over and done with.'' I detached myself. I knew it was wrong but I felt I deserved it. Although it hurt so much, it was nice that somebody did pay attention. I know that sounds sick, but that was how I felt then. It happened several times, whenever he could get a chance. I remember it happening, but I've learnt to block it out. I felt too ashamed to tell anybody. It was something I carried around myself. It was my problem. It ended when I was old enough to make a choice.'

The following quote regarding the effects of trauma captures a response to abuse which was expressed by several of the women interviewed in our research: 'Many individuals who have been traumatised do not want to feel anything. They have experienced intense and overwhelming feelings in the course of the trauma, and they have learned how to dampen or entirely cut them off. There are many ways to short-circuit feelings, such as alcohol and drug abuse, overwork or constant activity, or focus on physical symptoms and illness. Intense feelings that cannot be short-circuited often cannot be labelled and understood.'[11]

Curiously, sexually abused women reported no higher childhood rate of felt inferiority or helplessness than other women in the Sisters series.[12] They felt no more shame about their families than other women, presumably because much of the abuse was outside the nuclear family.[13] They also had only slightly higher rates of conduct problems than other children.[14] Yet we know these are potentially very damaging experiences, so we sought other responses in childhood which might reveal the type of emotional disturbance these children were prey to. We examined suicide attempts in childhood and found three times the rate: 17 per cent of those with 'marked' or 'moderate' sexual abuse had such attempts compared with 5 per cent of other children. We also examined self-harm in childhood and found that 13 per cent of those with sexual abuse compared with 4 per cent of other children exhibited behaviour such as cutting themselves with razor blades or scissors. This array of symptoms and personality problems seen following abuse is a well-known pattern of behaviour for survivors of trauma, and has been linked with the 'short-circuiting' of emotions described earlier.[15]

SEXUAL ABUSE AND ADULT DEPRESSION

In the Representative sample of mothers, women experiencing sexual abuse at 'marked' and 'moderate' levels of severity had the highest rate of depression of any abuse, with as many as half of the women being depressed in the year before interview.[16] In the Sisters series sexual abuse also related to a history of substance abuse: a third of those with sexual abuse had previous alcohol or drug abuse or dependence compared with 17 per cent of other women.[17] Again this has been identified as one of the ways in which abuse victims can 'shut off' their feelings concerning early trauma involving sexual abuse.

THE EXPERIENCE OF SISTERS

Obtaining corroborating accounts of sexual abuse from sisters was potentially a much harder task than that of corroborating other forms of neglect or abuse, not only because of the secrecy imposed by abusers but also because of the large proportion of abuse committed by perpetrators living outside the household. It was therefore expected that often an abuse would not be known about by a sister. Yet, when the association between sisters' accounts of abuse was examined there was a significant amount of agreement: 89 per cent of pairs agreed about the presence or absence of severe abuse in their own and each other's childhood.[18] When the abuses perpetrated by household member were considered separately they had a similar rate of agreement. However, as expected, there was little corroboration for abuse by non-household perpetrators, largely because the sister concerned rarely knew that the abuse had occurred.

The extent to which the sexual abuse was *experienced* by both sisters in a pair mirrored the corroboration result. Such shared experience in childhood was high for sexual abuse by a household member (92 per cent agreement) but low for non-household sexual abuse.[19] To put it simply: sisters gave particularly accurate accounts of each other's sexual abuses when the perpetrator lived in the household and the abuse could be witnessed by both. We found that in practice both daughters in the household tended to have been abused by the same person. When the sexual abuse was from a relative, family friend or stranger living outside the household it was more likely to occur to one sister alone. In these instances the other sister was less likely to know about it and report it at interview.

There were, however, a number of instances of both corroboration and concordance of sexual abuse by non-household members as shown in the following examples. One sister in a pair said about her abuser: 'He was married to a cousin of my father's. His wife was in hospital. He came to our house one afternoon and asked my mother if he could take me and my sister to the pictures. I was aged 12. He sat in the middle of us. He took my hand and had me rubbing his penis. I had gloves on. He took the glove off and made me use my hands. I kept pulling my hand away. It happened maybe six times.' On one occasion he locked her in the car and tried to take her clothes off. 'He told me I was a prick teaser. I was scared – petrified. I was frightened to pull my hand away. I didn't want my sister to know. I didn't tell anyone about it. I tried to avoid being alone with him where possible. One day we went back to his house. He came down and insisted on my sister going up to the front room to watch TV. He locked the kitchen door, undid his trousers and had me stroking him and whatever. I didn't kiss it, but he had me stroking it and rubbing it. He held me against the door pressing it.'

Her sister independently gave a similar account of her abuse by the same man: 'It was an uncle, married to my father's cousin, who used to try and interfere with us when we were children. He used to take my sister and me to the pictures and make us touch him. He used to sit one either side of him, our hands in his lap and we had to masturbate him. It happened three or four times when I was about seven. I didn't know what it was but I knew we shouldn't be doing it, that there was something not very nice about it. There were no words spoken, he'd just grab our hands. He stopped doing it to me, but carried on with my sister. She was very quiet as a child whereas he probably thought I might spill the beans. I remember being scared but feeling powerless – we didn't know what to do. We knew we shouldn't tell anyone, I don't know why. We kind of knew it would upset our mum, and my dad would go berserk, we'd better not say anything. After that he used to pick more on my sister, he tried it on with her until she was seventeen.'

CONCLUSION

From our exploration of sexual abuse, two important features emerge which need to be borne in mind for prevention and intervention. First, much sexual abuse is *not* from a natural father or even a relative but from family friends. Thus if a child is being sexually abused one cannot assume, as intervening agencies often do, that the father is necessarily the perpetrator. Second, the *Lolita* example given earlier emphasises the extreme predatory nature of many paedophiles. In the book Humbert describes hours spent in playgrounds watching 'nymphets' and being sexually aroused by chance contact with them. This is of course only one abusive scenario, but one which is possibly a greater danger to children since a single such character may abuse a large number of children. Many of the abused women we interviewed knew of sexual abuse to other children in the family, neighbourhood or school, committed by the same perpetrator.

The findings presented in this chapter mirror results gathered by another researcher in a rather different context. Michelle Eliot conducted a recent study involving interviews with nearly a hundred convicted sex offenders and showed a similar pattern to that reported here: one third of abuses were perpetrated by parents or step-parents who abused their own children, one third were known to their victims as family friends and one third were unknown to their victims.[20] All of the men interviewed had committed offences against more than one child, and a quarter had abused 10–40 children. Alarmingly, 7 per cent claimed they had each abused over 40 children.

A third of the men related how they frequented places where children went such as schools, shopping centres, playgrounds, parks, swimming baths and beaches. A third worked on being welcomed in the child's home, while 14 per cent 'took a chance' and touched the child when approached. A fifth of the men bribed their other victims to recruit new children. Two-thirds said the abuse took place in the offender's home and a third in the child's home. Nearly half admitted isolating their victims through babysitting.

One in eight of the offenders focused on innocent or trusting children and nearly half were attracted to children who seemed to lack confidence or had low self-esteem. The children seen as the most vulnerable were those who had family problems, were alone, lacked confidence, were pretty, trusting, young or small. The majority of the men had themselves been sexually abused in childhood. All committed their first offences as juveniles but the average age of first conviction was 31 years. Most said that the abuses became more serious over time.

The offenders ironically gave this advice to parents and teachers: to warn children of the dangers of secluded quiet places and playing alone particularly at night and near public toilets; to inform children that not all adults are trustworthy; to never accept lifts or talk to anyone who comes up to them, particularly a man alone; to encourage children to tell parents if anyone tries to trick them or make strange suggestions; to tell parents where they are going; and to always tell if someone is abusing them, even a friend. They recommended parents to be suspicious of anyone more interested in the children than the parents; to be aware of overly affectionate men; to be less trusting; to know that abusers will use any way to get to children; to teach children not to keep secrets and to tell children they have rights. Finally, they acknowledge single-parent families as good targets for paedophiles. This is the advice of 'experts', and as such should be taken seriously.

NOTES

1 Nabokov, V. (1959) *Lolita*, London: Weidenfeld and Nicolson (reprinted London: Penguin 1995).
2 Masson, J. (1984) *The Assault on Truth*, London: HarperCollins.
3 Department of Health and Social Security (1988) *Report of the Inquiry into Child Abuse in Cleveland*, London: HMSO.

At the time of writing the issue of whether the Cleveland children had in fact been abused has been reopened with additional evidence from social workers involved. This was reported in a Channel 4 television programme 'Death of Childhood' (27 May 1997). This suggested that the case originally reported in the media was distorted and that evidence over and above that provided by medical investigation of abuse of the children existed.

4 There is now a good deal of literature on false memory syndrome. The main proponents of this are: Loftus, E. and Ketcham, K. (1994) *The Myth of Repressed Memory*, New York: St Martin's Press.

The main antagonists of this view are: Herman, H. and Schatzow, M. (1987) 'Recovery and verification of memories of childhood sexual trauma', *Psychoanalytic Psychology* 4: 1–14.

5 For definitions of abuse and review see Finkelhor, D.A. (1986) *Sourcebook on Child Sexual Abuse*, California: Sage Publications.
6 For a review of sexual abuse studies see Gillham, B. (1991) *The Facts about Child Sexual Abuse*, London: Cassell Educational Ltd.
7 Prevalence of contact sexual abuse in the Representative London Women series was 9% (25/286).
8 In the Representative London Women series, the prevalence of sexual abuse for the total number of different household arrangements in childhood (N = 465) was 4% (10/282) for families headed by both natural parents and 5% (3/65) where a lone parent was responsible for the child. This compared with 11% (3/27) for parent and step-parent arrangements and 9% (8/91) of other arrangements including institutions and living with relatives or friends but without a natural parent (p < 0.05).
9 *Table 6.1* Sexual abuse and other abuses (Representative London Women series) (% sexual abuse)

Other abuse	Present	Absent	
Neglect	32 (16/50)	4 (9/236)	p < 0.001
Physical abuse	23 (12/52)	6 (13/234)	p < 0.001
Antipathy from mother	16 (8/50)	7 (17/236)	NS
Antipathy from father	9 (5/56)	9 (20/230)	NS

10 In the Sisters series there were 46 women with at least one severe abuse, and if multiples are included then a total of 59 different severe abuses by different perpetrators were recorded. Imposed secretiveness was reported in the Sisters series for 34% (20) of all severe abuses. Confiding (even to low levels) about sexual abuse was 17% (10). Official contact concerning sexual abuse in the Sisters series was 7% (4) of all severe abuses.

11 Allen, J. (1995) *Coping with Trauma*, Washington: American Psychiatric Press Inc.

12 *Table 6.2* Sexual abuse, childhood self-esteem and coping (Sisters series)

Sexual abuse	% inferiority	% helplessness
Present	50 (23/46)	24 (11/46)
Absent	53 (81/152)	16 (24/152)
	NS	NS

13 *Table 6.3* Sexual abuse and childhood relations to others (Sisters series)

Sexual abuse	% shame	% loneliness
Present	50 (23/46)	50 (23/46)
Absent	41 (63/152)	35 (53/152)
	NS	NS

14 *Table 6.4* Sexual abuse and disturbance in childhood (Sisters series)

Sexual abuse	% conduct problems	% suicide attempt	% self-harm behaviour
Present	11 (5/46)	17 (8/46)	13 (6/46)
Absent	7 (10/152)	5 (7/152)	4 (6/152)
	NS	p < 0.025	p < 0.10

15 Herman, J. (1992) *Trauma and Recovery*, London: Pandora; USA: Basic Books.

16 Among women with childhood sexual abuse in the Representative series 52% (13/25) became depressed versus 14% (37/261) of remaining women, p < 0.001

For full results see Bifulco, A., Brown, G.W. and Adler, Z. (1991) 'Early sexual abuse and clinical depression in adult life', *British Journal of Psychiatry 159*: 115–122.

17 *Table 6.5* Sexual abuse and life-time substance abuse (Sisters series)

Sexual abuse	% substance abuse
Present	33 (15/46)
Absent	17 (26/152)
	$p < 0.05$

18 Agreement between sisters for the occurrence of any sexual abuse was 0.52 (Kw, $p < 0.0001$) with 89% of pairs in agreement. For sexual abuse by household members the correlation was 0.56 (Kw, $p < 0.0001$) with 98% of pairs in agreement. For abuse by non-household members the correlation was 0.37 (Kw, $p < 0.01$) with 89% of pairs in agreement.

19 Eighty-six per cent of sister pairs both suffered sexual abuse, with a correlation of 0.27 (Kw, $p < 0.001$). For sexual abuse by a household member the concordance was much higher with 92% of pairs having similar abuse and the correlation being 0.56 (Kw, $p < 0.0001$). There was no similarity in sisters' experience for abuse by non-household member (correlation of 0.15, NS).

20 Eliot, M. (1995) 'Child sexual abuse prevention: what offenders tell us', *Child Abuse and Neglect 19*: 579–594.

Chapter 7

Psychological abuse: hostage to fortune

Captivity, which brings the victim into prolonged contact with the perpetrator, creates a special type of relationship, one of coercive control. This is equally true whether the victim is taken captive entirely by force, as in the case of prisoners and hostages, or by a combination of force, intimidation, and enticement, as in the case of religious cult members, battered women and abused children. The psychological impact of subordination to coercive control may have many common features, whether the subordination occurs within the public sphere of politics or within the private sphere of sexual and domestic relations.

(Herman 1994: 74–75)[1]

Forcing a child to bathe in ice-cold water; making a bed-wetter sleep on the same urine-soaked sheets for weeks; threatening to withhold life-sustaining medication from a sick child: these are some of the examples of sadistic parental behaviour recounted in the course of our research surveys. Although elements of neglect and other abuse often featured in such examples, there was a distinctively callous quality to these experiences which we felt merited a new classification. The category of psychological abuse was thus added only recently to our taxonomy of childhood maltreatment.

In previous chapters the context within which neglect or abuse occurred showed that in many instances the mistreatment could be understood in relation to problematic family circumstances and the strain endured by parents. Psychological abuse, by comparison, involved harming a child in a far more calculated way which was difficult to comprehend in terms of poor parenting skills or difficult circumstances. While a rejecting remark made in the heat of the moment or smacks from an exasperated parent are within many parent's experience, psychological abuse encompassed parental behaviours which most would consider unthinkable, typically involving extreme levels of control, domination and denigration.

DEFINING PSYCHOLOGICAL ABUSE

Domination of the child was considered a key characteristic in defining this category of abuse. Arguably, domination features in all forms of abuse. However, what distinguishes psychological abuse from others is the means by which this aim is achieved. Physical hitting and sexual contact are absent, although sometimes they occur in parallel to increase the fear inculcated. In their place are callous actions or words, often premeditated and enjoyed by the perpetrator. They range from casual humiliations to extreme cases of degradation.

Our category of psychological abuse approximates to the NSPCC's category of 'emotional abuse', which they define as 'the severe adverse effect on the behaviour and emotional development of a child caused by persistent or severe emotional ill-treatment or rejection'.[2] However, this definition potentially confounds the nature of the abuse with its effects. For the purposes of our research it was important to distinguish the *characteristics* of the ill-treatment from their *effect* upon the child. We had to avoid the tautological trap of defining psychological abuse as that which causes psychological damage, a characteristic which has been shown to be common to all abuse. Thus, we defined psychological abuse in terms of the perpetrator's actions rather than their impact on the child. It was the *potential* for psychological harm which was considered pertinent rather than the level of actual psychological injury incurred by the child. This approach was consistent with our method of defining other types of neglect and abuse. Our definition of physical abuse, for example, takes into account the force and frequency of blows delivered and their likelihood of causing injury rather than the extent of actual physical or emotional injury to the child.

TYPES OF PSYCHOLOGICAL ABUSE

Developing a system for grading examples of psychological abuse proved complex because of the diversity of perpetrators' techniques and behaviours. Very different experiences seemed to us to be equally severe and deserving of classification. For example, locking a terrified child in a dark cellar, humiliating a child in front of other adults, forcing a child to steal, or promising some treat only to have it rescinded at the last moment – all seemed to be different forms of a similar cynical manipulation.

Four distinct means of gaining domination over a child were identified as falling under the umbrella of psychological abuse. Each seemed to mirror a type of abuse already defined in earlier chapters but with an added sadistic element. The first involved depriving the child of basic physical or emotional needs, and was akin to neglect. However, it also involved an element of toying with the child's feelings and using conscious strategies to deprive the child of food, light, sleep or companionship in order to induce submission. A second form of psychological abuse involved inflicting distress, terror or humiliation, and was allied to physical abuse, but used a more mental form of torture rather than physical force to achieve compliance. A third type of psychological abuse had similarities with antipathy, and involved threats of abandonment and destroying the child's sense of worth and identity. The fourth type of psychological abuse concerned the use of emotional blackmail and corruption of the child, and occurred most commonly with sexual abuse. Each category of psychological abuse was rated separately for severity under the usual 'marked', 'moderate' and 'mild' scoring system. Taking these different subscales into account, an overall level of psychological abuse was derived using the same scaling method.

DEPRIVATION OF PHYSICAL AND EMOTIONAL NEEDS

The first subcategory of psychological abuse, namely deprivation of needs, was demonstrated by behaviours such as locking a child in a cold, dark room with minimal food and clothing for hours at a time. Such extreme examples warranted a 'marked' rating. This deprivation exceeded neglect as defined in earlier chapters because of the conscious strategy of the parent in withholding basic resources from the child with the intention of domination. The perpetrator typically isolated and stigmatised the child using dehumanising treatment. This maltreatment contrasts with 'simple' neglect where children are ignored by parents rather than being made the focus of such control.

Examples of 'moderate' deprivation of basic needs included children whose parents enforced isolation on them by forbidding them from playing or conversing with their friends or siblings. One example involved a father locking away all his daughter's clothes except for her school uniform and a plastic mac when she wanted to go out to a club with her friends on a Saturday afternoon, thus preventing her from going. 'Mild' examples in this category involved a child who was made to sit rigid on a chair facing a wall for long periods of time as punishment.

Sometimes psychological abuse involved a more focused form of deprivation which occurred when children had a valued possession taken away and destroyed in a callous manner. Often the object in question was a toy, present, pet or some object of comfort. A 'marked' example was recounted by a women who was looked after by her aunt: 'I was about nine, and I had a pet dog. My aunt picked me up from school after we had been away on a trip for a few days. She handed me the dog's collar and lead and said, "You won't be needing these any more – the dog's dead." My aunt had the dog put down. It was the first thing she said as I got off the coach.' Not only was the act of destroying the child's pet unnecessarily cruel, but the cold manner and premeditated timing in telling the child were particularly callous. For these reasons this was considered a prime example of psychological abuse. We heard of other incidents involving pets, including one girl's father who made her witness him killing, cooking and eating her pet rabbits.

A case which clearly demonstrated the destruction of a valued object relating to the child's sense of identity was the example of the neglected child whose stepmother ripped up the only photograph of her dead mother that the child possessed. This was similar to an account of a stepfather who destroyed a child's small wooden cot given to her by her father before he died. The stepfather smashed it up in front of the child, stamped on it and ritually burned it in the garden.

INFLICTING PHYSICAL PAIN, TERRORISING OR HUMILIATING

Psychological abuse also showed itself in incidents involving the infliction of marked physical discomfort by means other than hitting, such as being forced to eat indigestible food. Several women told us of the way meal times were used as punishment. A number of parents went to unreasonable lengths in forcing their children to eat an entire meal. An example of 'moderate' abuse was a father who insisted that his child finished everything on her plate at each meal. When she was unable to, he kept bringing the same plate of food back to her cold at every meal time until nothing was left on the plate. Often she vomited trying to finish it.

Another abusive technique involved terrorising the child and playing on the child's natural fears. Common examples of this form of abuse, rated as 'moderate' in severity, involved forcing a child known to be petrified of the dark, to remain locked in a darkened room. A 'mild' example was provided by a woman who described her stepmother as vindictive: 'She used to make me clean daddy-long-legs out of the house when she knew that I was terrified of them.'

Some parents psychologically abused their children by using degrading words or actions to induce feelings of shame. A common theme running through many of these examples of humiliation was the use of natural body functions as a vehicle for parental cruelty. Eating, sleeping, urinating and defecating featured regularly. 'Marked' examples involved accounts of incontinent children having their faces wiped in urine-soaked sheets as punishment for bed-wetting, and one child whose head was pushed into faeces. One woman recounted the ridicule she experienced for her incontinence: 'They used to call me a baby when I wet myself. Once when I was about ten they made me wear a nappy to go to the shops.' Others were forced to wear unclean, stinking underwear for weeks at a time. Such ridicule only served to heighten the child's anxiety and further aggravate their bed-wetting problem.

Sometimes the humiliation relied on the presence of others to induce feelings of degradation. An example of this 'public' form of humiliation was that of a teenage girl at boarding school who was forced to shower and sleep in a separate room from her classmates after the discovery by teachers that she was a lesbian. This differential treatment was carried out in the public arena to inflict the maximum possible potential for shame. A similar example at a 'moderate' level was the case of a mother who spread false stories about her daughter being a thief so that the girl was never trusted by others in the small community where they lived. 'Mild' forms of such abuse involved verbal threats which were never actually carried out. For example, one mother threatened to take her incontinent daughter's urine-soaked sheets to school to parade at assembly but never actually did so.

ABANDONMENT AND DISORIENTATION

Psychological abuse also involved extreme rejection, whereby the child was wished either dead or out of existence. 'Marked' examples included the comments one girl's mother made to her: 'Mother frequently wished me dead. She said she wished the milk she had fed me as a baby had choked me. As a teenager, when I survived my first suicide attempt her first words to me were "Do it right next time."' Threats of abandonment also featured. A 'moderate' example which happened to a woman and her siblings when she was only five years old was the following: 'I don't know what we were doing wrong but mother made us all sit on stools and she told us that we'd been bad and we were to sit there because the men were coming to take us away to the "bad girls' home". Then, unbeknown to us, she got our dad to go outside and ring the doorbell and pretend he was the policeman. It gave me a terrible fright, being so young at the time.'

Instilling mental confusion or disorientation was another form of psychological abuse imposed on children. A state of bewilderment was induced by invalidating the reality of the child's senses. A 'marked' example was suffered by a girl who was repeatedly given instructions which were then promptly countermanded. On one occasion she was ordered to hang and re-hang washing over a period of an hour, during which time she was told repeatedly that she had misheard the instructions. On another occasion she was forced to clean the family's shoes and then promptly reclean them. This strategy undermined the child's ability to believe the evidence of her own senses – she was never sure whether she had heard her stepfather correctly. Prolonged use of this disorientation technique led to children feeling that they were losing their sanity, as the girl describes: 'It would go on for so many days and so many weeks that you began to wonder whether you were going mad, whether you were actually losing control of yourself because he was making you feel as though you had misunderstood the first command or that you had done the opposite of what he'd asked.' Another example involved convincing the child that she had no memory of her natural father whom she had lost when aged eight. As an adult, the woman insisted that she could not recall her father and yet, when probed, was able to give a detailed description of her childhood relationship with him. An example of 'mild' disorienting abuse was to promise a treat only to rescind it once the child was about to receive it.

EMOTIONAL BLACKMAIL AND CORRUPTION

Another type of abuse used to exert control over children was that of emotional blackmail whereby threats to others' safety were made to elicit compliance. The child would thus be so fearful of the consequence that compliance with any of the abuser's demands was guaranteed. This form of psychological abuse most commonly accompanied sexual abuse. A 'marked' example involved the case of a woman whose father threatened to beat her brothers and sisters if she did not comply with his sexual demands. These threats constituted psychological abuse in addition to sexual abuse, and added considerably to her trauma. Another teenager had her handbag containing details of her address stolen by the stranger who raped her. He threatened to find her and kill her if she told the police about the rape.

One form of psychological abuse encountered relatively rarely in our surveys was that of corruption or exploitation. This category involved placing the child in a situation were her moral welfare was at risk, such as being made to steal, being pictured for pornographic material or forced into prostitution. One example involved a pair of sisters who were recruited by a paedophile ring. Another example included in this category involved a girl from an affluent but neglectful home. She was introduced to drugs by her mother who told her to taste some 'sherbet'. This was in fact amphetamine and the child subsequently developed a drug habit.

PREVALENCE OF PSYCHOLOGICAL ABUSE

Psychological abuse was the rarest abuse encountered in our samples. This was the case even in our series of sisters, half of whom were selected for the presence of other types of neglect and abuse. Only 8 per cent in the Sisters series experienced psychological abuse to 'marked' or 'moderate' levels, with a further 7 per cent rated as experiencing it in a 'mild' form.[3] It was not possible to ascertain figures for the prevalence of psychological abuse among the Representative London Women series since it was not measured at the time that series was studied. However, its rarity is suggested by the presence of only one severe ('marked' or 'moderate') example (1 per cent) in the *unselected* part of the Sisters series. Also in this group 'mild' psychological abuse was encountered in only 3 per cent of women.

In terms of reported cases, figures from the NSPCC show that emotional abuse formed the reason for placing children on the risk register in only 2 per cent of cases between 1988 and 1990.[4] Its low incidence partly reflects the substantial overlap between this form of abuse and others. Under national procedures for reporting abuse, cases where it is present are usually categorised in terms of the accompanying forms of abuse such as sexual or physical, which are more readily identifiable. The category of emotional abuse is thus used as a reason for registering a child only if it is the sole form of abuse occurring. Hence arriving at an estimate of the size of the problem using the number of reported cases of psychological abuse is uninformative. The low rate of known cases of psychological abuse may also be due to difficulties in its categorisation. Psychological abuse can involve a host of disparate actions, the effects of which are mostly invisible. Physical or sexual abuse, by comparison, involves specific delineable actions on the part of the perpetrator, and can often be proved by forensic or medical tests.

PERPETRATORS OF PSYCHOLOGICAL ABUSE

Perpetrators of the abuse were equally mothers or fathers, natural or surrogate. However, the rarity of the experience made it difficult to describe the features of families or situations in which it was more common. We were under the impression that psychological abuse arose mainly as a function of characteristics of the perpetrator in terms of sadistic tendencies rather than as a function of characteristics of the particular child or family type. In some step-families, it seemed that step-parents were concerned to eradicate the child's efforts to identify with their predecessor, the child's natural parent. In other situations it could be seen as an example of over-intrusive and zealous parenting as in the case of a father who forced his daughter to memorise and recite numerous pages of the dictionary, repeating each page for weeks at a time until her recitation was perfect.

THE CONTEXT OF PSYCHOLOGICAL ABUSE

We have already described how psychological abuse at times existed in conjunction with sexual or physical abuse, in the sense that the two behaviours were intertwined. However, even among the remaining independent abuses, all instances of psychological abuse were found to occur within the context of a home environment characterised by antipathy, neglect, physical or sexual abuse.[5] It was strongly associated with physical abuse and neglect in particular: all but one individual with psychological abuse experienced physical abuse and all but three suffered parental neglect.

An example of the way in which sexual abuse could be paralleled with intermittent psychological abuse by the same perpetrator is the story of *Lolita* described in the last chapter. Psychologically abusive techniques were used to misinform the child about the consequences she faced following any disclosure of the sexual abuse. Psychological manipulation increased her terror so that remaining with the sexual abuser was seen as the less frightening option. Such psychologically abusive methods are evident in the predatory techniques of paedophiles when isolating a child and 'grooming' them to be acquiescent in the abuse.

Sometimes psychological abuse followed on as a consequence of a child disclosing another type of abuse. For example, one woman told us how she was sexually abused by her mother's boyfriend. At the age of eleven she plucked up the courage to tell her mother about the abuse. The mother confronted her boyfriend about it, only to be told by him that the girl had seduced him against his wishes. The mother chose to believe her boyfriend, and moved him into the household as the children's new stepfather. Thereafter the mother continued to ignore the child and instead poured her energies into the relationship with her boyfriend. In adulthood the woman reflected that she found her mother's response more damaging than the original sexual abuse had been.

In another case described in previous chapters, the detection of a father's physical abuse by a child's teacher ultimately led to a switch to psychological abuse as an alternative. The teacher alerted social services to the possibility of the physical abuse, but their investigation failed to substantiate the allegations. To evade detection the father reverted increasingly to psychological techniques of abusing his daughter, thus leaving no physical marks which might be detected by the authorities.

SECRETIVENESS OF PSYCHOLOGICAL ABUSE

Psychological abuse tends to be unrecognised by society at large because of its complex definition and subtle, multi-faceted expression. While most people have a reasonable understanding of what constitutes physical and sexual abuse, the identification of psychological abuse remains more illusive. This is partly the reason why the children themselves often failed to alert the outside world to this form of maltreatment. To confide would require a full exposition of the context, as one woman explained: 'How could I tell anyone my stepfather made me take the washing out and then bring it in again, or polish the shoes more than once. They simply wouldn't see anything very bad in that. It was so difficult to describe what it was like. It would have been easier to say I'd been hit.'

When one woman attempted to tell an aunt about her father's severe psychological abuse of her and her sisters, her father's actions were dismissed as merely quirky or odd rather than abusive, and consequently the abuse continued unabated. The research interview was the first occasion on which she had been given the chance to recount fully her childhood experience and to express the emotional pain she had suffered at the time. She harboured deep resentment towards her father but also to her aunt whom she held responsible for prolonging her childhood misery by failing to take her disclosure of abuse seriously.

CHILDHOOD COPING AND SELF-ESTEEM

Sometimes anger served to motivate abused children to seek ways of re-establishing their identity and dignity. One girl who suffered marked abuse at the hands of her stepfather described her need to exercise choice and control. Despite the utter hopelessness of her particular situation, she tried to devise a means of taking control: 'I had to fight him somehow. I had to stop him from doing it. I tried to stop him in any way, shape or form.' She would, for instance, put on a brave face and pretend that she was unaffected by the deprivation to which he subjected her in order to get revenge. 'When he looked in the door and expected to see me lying there crying, I'd sit and smile at him. I began to give him back what he did to me, I let him see that he wasn't getting to me.' This battle of wills was the only means she had at her disposal for countering the psychological abuse. She continued to use these techniques, even though at times she received further mistreatment or was beaten for her defiance.

Holding on to one's sense of reality and retaining any sense of self-worth are extraordinarily difficult when faced with extreme psychological maltreatment. Children who experienced psychological abuse showed a higher rate of felt inferiority with as many as 80 per cent having such low self-esteem in childhood.[6] There was also some evidence they tended to suffer more shame, and loneliness than other children.[7]

Psychologically abused children also showed signs of disturbance similar to that experienced by the sexually abused children described in the last chapter. They were four times more likely to try to commit suicide in childhood (27 per cent versus 6 per cent of other children) and eight times more likely to describe self-harming behaviour in childhood (33 per cent versus 4 per cent).[8] Often children were shown little sympathy for such acts, as this girl's experience shows: 'First I tried to cut myself with a safety pin when I was around thirteen or fourteen. Then I tried it with razor blades. That's when my brother told my dad. Dad said "If you're going to do that sort of thing, do it outside – I don't want blood all over my home." I felt so hurt.'

PSYCHOLOGICAL ABUSE AND ADULT DISORDER

Showing an association of psychological abuse with adult depression is made difficult by its rarity and by its lack of independence from other abuses. However, in the Sisters series, although it showed a relationship to depression, this was no higher than among those with other forms of neglect or abuse. Thus 27 per cent of those with psychological abuse were depressed in the year of interview compared with 35 per cent of those with neglect, physical or sexual abuse and 13 per cent of those with no abuse.[9] We therefore additionally examined prior suicide attempts in adulthood to continue with a possible alternative diagnosis of self-harm as discussed in the last chapter. This proved to be highly related, with 53 per cent of those with psychological abuse having made a suicide attempt in early adult life compared with 20 per cent of those without.[10] (Of course the latter figure would include women with sexual and other abuse.) As with sexual abuse, there was also some evidence that these women had a higher rate of prior episodes of alcohol or drug abuse: 40 per cent of them reported such an episode in their adult lives compared with 19 per cent of other women.

PSYCHOLOGICAL ABUSE IN ADULTHOOD

In many respects the experience of children dominated by psychologically abusing parents echoes that of women who are dominated by controlling partners in adulthood. This is particularly the case within the context of domestic violence. A recent report by NCH Action for Children documenting the experience of mothers in violent relationships illustrated the controlling behaviours to which they were subjected at the hands of their domineering partners.[11] These included enforced confinement with severe limitations on freedom of movement, and limited access to financial resources. More than two-fifths of these women were reported to have been locked in their own homes, and more than a fifth had their clothes taken away. The majority were subjected to repeated insults and humiliations in front of others. The women were often forbidden friendships or other external sources of social support which might validate their feelings of self-worth and identity and provide them with a measure of independence.

Such methods of coercive control are not restricted to situations of violent adult relationships or child abuse. Similar methods of domination have been reportedly used in the induction of women into prostitution, where the technique is known as 'seasoning'. This method 'is meant to break its victim's will, reduce her ego and separate her from her previous life. All procuring strategies include some form of seasoning. . . . Seasoning inculcates dependence and indebtedness in the victim.'[12] Such techniques have been described as brain-washing, aimed at creating a permanent personality change in the victim.[13] The process has been encapsulated as 'unfreezing', 'changing' and 'refreezing' of the victim's psychological processes so that she ultimately integrates and articulates changes in her values, attitudes and beliefs in line with that of the perpetrator.

CAPTOR AND CAPTIVE

Several writers have drawn parallels between the process of domination that occurs in the domestic arena and that which occurs in the political arena. A number of oppressive contexts have been identified in which psychological abuse akin to brain-washing occurs: 'concentration camps; hostage situations; political prisoners; forced labour camps; violently isolative religious cults . . . some forms of child abuse . . . thought reform prisons; female sexual slavery, including forced prostitution and prolonged woman-battering'.[14] The quote at the beginning of this chapter similarly links the abuse of children and women in domestic situations with that experienced by political hostages.

Many are now familiar with accounts of the treatment political hostages are subjected to, notably after the series of books published by the ex-Beirut hostages in the early 1990s relating their years held captive by Shi'ite militiamen. They recount the way in which their captors callously toyed with their emotions, perceptions and physical needs in order to achieve complete submission. They also describe the complex relationship that can emerge between captor and captive where, as in childhood, enforced dependency on a brutal provider significantly damages the victim's belief in themselves and their ability to form relationships with others thereafter.

We collected childhood histories in our interviews which at times bore striking similarities to the accounts of such captivity – dramas played out in the homes of British families not Middle Eastern war zones. One particular example shared similarities with an account of captivity given by the former Beirut hostage Brian Keenan. In his book *An Evil Cradling*, he recounts his experiences of being held in a number of makeshift prison cells in appalling conditions.[15] Typically each cramped cell contained nothing but a stinking mattress on the floor. Personal possessions were removed: the clothes he stood up in were all he possessed. He was given no extra clothing despite freezing weather conditions at times. For much of the time he was held with no light source, in total darkness. He was fed only one meal a day, consisting of bread, jam and an egg. He survived like this, or in similar conditions, for over five years. In that time he was also subjected to several savage beatings.

Keenan's account was reminiscent of one of the most extreme examples of psychological abuse which emerged in the course of our research. It involved a woman whose stepfather took a ferocious dislike to her as a child, fuelled by her comments about preferring to live with her 'real' father. She was brutally punished for such behaviour. For several days at a time she would be locked in her room, clothed only in a nightdress. The room was stripped of anything which might afford her comfort, such as toys or personal possessions. Her stepfather had removed the blankets, curtains and lightbulb, leaving only a bare mattress. She received only one meagre meal per day, made up of a sandwich and some biscuits. Her stepfather also periodically beat her using his belt on her back until she bled from the wounds. She was only aged eight when this treatment began.

Keenan's experience as a hostage and the girl's account of childhood demonstrate close parallels. Basic physical needs were ignored, and further psychological abuse was inflicted by the removal of personal possessions to additionally strip the individual of a sense of identity. The knowledge that even worse treatment would follow if any attempt was make at retaliation paralysed them into submission. In each instance the strategies used by their captors were strikingly similar, and their aim the same – total domination. These examples serve to illustrate that techniques used to enforce submission are not restricted to child victims but can occur in various exploitative situations. In later chapters we consider how neglect and abuse in general can also define a woman's context in adult life.

CONCLUSION

Psychological abuse is a relatively new area of study for investigators of childhood experience. Although we know relatively little about the true impact of such abusive behaviour, we can assume it is a potent factor, and certainly deserving of more substantial investigation. Further study is required to establish its prevalence in the community at large and its presence also needs to be assessed in the childhood experiences of particular populations such as psychiatric in-patients, female offenders and the homeless, where we would hypothesise that its prevalence is high.

When we began our first childhood research twenty years ago it was sparked by the investigation of the impact of loss of a parent, which led to the study of neglect. Since then we have witnessed a gradual emergence of various new features of childhood maltreatment. If neglect and loss of mother were the focus of study in the 1970s and physical and sexual abuse in the 1980s, it is psychological abuse that is likely to be seen in the future as the contribution of the studies of the 1990s. While the identification of psychological abuse marks the latest evolution of our own assessments of childhood experience, we also hope it is the last, and that by the millennium the research community will have finally documented all the varieties of childhood abuse to be uncovered.

NOTES

1 Herman, J. (1994) *Trauma and Recovery*, London: Pandora Books.
2 Report of the National Commission of Inquiry into the Prevention of Child Abuse (1996) *Childhood Matters*, London: The Stationery Office.

3   Fifteen of the women in the Sisters series (8%) had psychological abuse at 'marked' or 'moderate' levels, and a further 7% (13) had 'mild' psychological abuse. In the unselected Sisters series only 1% (1/80) experienced severe psychological abuse, and 3% (2/80) experienced it to a 'mild' level.

4   Creighton, S. (1992) *Child Abuse Trends in England and Wales 1988–90*, London: NSPCC.

5   *Table 7.1* Overlap of psychological abuse with other abuses (Sisters series) (% psychological abuse)

	Other abuse		
	Present	Absent	
Sexual abuse	22 (10/46)	3 (5/152)	$p < 0.005$
Physical abuse	18 (14/79)	1 (1/119)	$p < 0.001$
Neglect	23 (12/53)	2 (3/145)	$p < 0.001$
Antipathy from mother	14 (10/69)	4 (5/129)	$p < 0.025$
Antipathy from father	11 (4/38)	7 (11/160)	NS

6   *Table 7.2* Psychological abuse self-esteem and coping in childhood (Sisters series)

Psychological abuse	% felt inferiority	% helpless
Present	80 (12/15)	27 (4/15)
Absent	50 (92/183)	17 (31/183)
	$p < 0.10$	NS

7   *Table 7.3* Psychological abuse and relations to others (Sisters series)

Psychological abuse	% felt shame	% felt loneliness
Present	73 (11/15)	53 (8/15)
Absent	41 (75/183)	37 (68/183)
	$p < 0.05$	NS

8   *Table 7.4* Psychological abuse and disturbance in childhood (Sisters series)

Psychological abuse	% suicide attempt	% self-harm behaviour
Present	27 (4/15)	33 (5/15)
Absent	6 (11/183)	4 (7/183)
	$p < 0.025$	$p < 0.001$

9   *Table 7.5* Psychological abuse and depression (Sisters series)

	% depressed
Psychological abuse	27 (4/15)
Other neglect/abuse	35 (33/94)
Neither	13 (12/89)
	$p < 0.005$

10   *Table 7.6* Psychological abuse and other adult disorder (Sisters series)

Psychological abuse	% prior suicide attempt	% substance abuse
Present	53 (8/15)	40 (6/15)
Absent	20 (36/183)	19 (35/183)
	$p < 0.01$	$p < 0.10$

11 NCH Action for Children (1994) *The Hidden Victims: Children and Domestic Violence*, London: NCH Action for Children.
12 Barry, K. (1981) *Female Sexual Slavery*, New York: Avon Books.
13 Okun, L. (1986) *Woman Abuse. Facts Replacing Myths*, Albany: State University of New York Press.
14 Ibid.
15 Keenan, B. (1993) *An Evil Cradling*, London: Vintage edition, Random House.

Part III

Contexts and outcomes

The final section of this book aims to broaden the discussion of childhood neglect and abuse to take account both of the childhood family context in which it occurs and the adult sequelae which render an individual susceptible to later depressive disorder. First we examine the effect of multiple forms of adversity in childhood to assess whether this increases the risk of adult depression. We do this by examining the effects of experiencing *more* than one type of abuse over one alone and also by examining the effects of other childhood difficulties such as family poverty or parental psychiatric disorder to see if these add to the risk of adult depression.

Second, we explore the types of experiences which link maltreatment in childhood with vulnerability to depression in later adult life. We examine adult violence and sexual assault towards the women to see if their effects parallel childhood abuse by increasing depressive risk. We also examine adult vulnerability factors such as low self-esteem and poor support, and assess the role they perform in increasing risk of depression when life crises are encountered.

Finally, we explore the possible *protective* effects of various experiences throughout the life course, which may decrease risk of either adult vulnerability or subsequent depression. Since this topic is still under investigation in the team's current research projects, we highlight factors which seem *at present* to be likely candidates as protective factors against depression. Although further research and analysis is required to provide a more complete picture, we hope that the inclusion of positive as well as negative experiences portrays a less fatalistic interpretation of the link between childhood experience and adult depression.

Chapter 8

Multiple adversities: stressful family contexts

A variety of studies have shown that, on the whole, single stressful experiences that occur truly in isolation carry rather low psychosocial risks. Serious risks tend to occur from the *combination* of adversities or stressors occurring at the same time, from meaningful links between a current stress and a previous adversity, or from accumulations of stresses/adversities over time.

(Caprara and Rutter 1995: 42)[1]

The previous chapters have examined six separate types of childhood maltreatment reflecting aspects of neglect and abuse. While for the purposes of this book they have been presented as separate categories of experience, in reality they may, and often do, coincide. What is more, they typically occur in the context of other challenging conditions which may play a role in escalating risk for depression, such as parental separation or poverty. In this chapter we examine the effects of both multiple abuse in childhood and the possible role played by associated factors involving the wider family environment.

To illustrate the broader family context in which childhood neglect or abuse occurs we begin by considering one woman's unhappy childhood. She experienced many of the types of maltreatment discussed in earlier chapters in combination with a disruptive family life. Her difficulties began when her parents separated shortly after her birth. Her mother couldn't cope alone with the children and abandoned them to social services: 'Mother took myself and two older sisters down to the local authority and apparently she said to my eldest sister ''Just look after your sisters for a little while, I'll only be half an hour'', and that was it, she never came back. My father wasn't around anywhere, nobody knew where he was. So they had no alternative but to place us in care.'

She and her sisters spent five years in a children's home and then returned to their father after he remarried, to a woman much younger than himself. This father was extremely authoritarian and distant. The stepmother, in her early twenties, was unable to cope with the three children she inherited on marrying. The child was neglected: neither parent took any interest in how she was doing at school, they discouraged her from bringing friends to the house, and never demonstrated any sympathy towards her. Their uncaring attitude showed itself when the child was unwell: 'I remember when I was eleven I was very ill. I remember having to scream in order to be taken to the hospital. On another occasion I got knocked down by a car and slightly hurt and father actually hit me for getting run over. He wasn't worried about the fact I'd been run over, he was more worried about the fact I'd ruined my new jeans and I'd taken so long to come home.'

There was no closeness or warmth from either parent: 'I think only once did dad attempt to give me a kiss or a cuddle. I remember detesting him from the time he told me that my real mother hadn't wanted me. He made me feel extremely unloved and unlovable because my real mum was the obvious person who should have loved me and didn't, and he obviously didn't love me either.' Her father used to beat her on a regular basis, to the extent that she was frightened to go home after school. She was also sexually abused. 'I was ten when it happened with my grandad, my stepmother's father. It happened several times, whenever he got the chance.'

There were other family problems. Her father gambled compulsively and left the family short of money, which led to arguments with his wife. 'They were always arguing. You'd be on edge from the minute you got up. There was always tension in the house – the only time you felt safe was when it was bedtime.' There were several brief separations when her father left home and stepmother was left alone with his children. The father's gambling led to other difficulties: 'He hadn't been paying the rent. We were evicted about three times and had to go and live in bed and breakfast places.'

COMBINATIONS OF ABUSE

In this example we see how a child can experience neglect and abuse from several perpetrators simultaneously. This woman suffered neglect from her father and stepmother, both of whom seemed too distracted by their own problems to care for her. Subsequently she was exposed to physical abuse from her father and sexual abuse from her grandfather. Previous chapters have illustrated the high association between each of these different forms of neglect and abuse and the complex situations in which they arise. In order to undertake further analysis of childhood experience, particularly in terms of a range of later adult experience, we found it useful to devise a more compact assessment of early experience. We were looking for a 'shorthand' method of summarising what constituted an abusive childhood. It proved possible to consider different forms of abuse as equivalent because each had been assessed in an identical manner, and rated on a four-point scale of severity, with all proving consistent in their relationship with depression. Thus we could contrast those with at least one such experience with those without, as well as examining the effects of multiple abuse in childhood.

When we examined combinations of all six types of maltreatment outlined in previous chapters in relation to adult depression, it was the experience of neglect *or* physical abuse *or* sexual abuse which provided, at least in a statistical sense, the most economical coverage of all the negative experiences. The remaining experiences were either so rare (such as psychological abuse), or so closely tied to another factor (such as role-reversal to neglect), or overlapped so much with more than one other factor (such as antipathy overlapping with neglect and physical abuse) that in practice only the three experiences were required to represent the best summary of all six. This enabled us to simplify our analysis so that women's childhoods could be described in terms of their experience of at least one of these three abuses. With this compact assessment we were then able to examine the prevalence and the effects of at least *one* experience of abuse in our series compared to combinations of these.

In the Representative London Women sample of working-class mothers, 29 per cent proved to have suffered at least *one* experience of neglect, physical or sexual abuse in childhood. In the unselected part of the Sisters series (which unlike the Representative series included middle-class women and single women without children), the rate was around 20 per cent. Thus the presence of at least one such abusive experience can be seen to be relatively common, with around a quarter of women in the community being affected. Multiple abuse in terms of *two* or more different types of maltreatment during childhood was experienced by 12 per cent of the Representative London Women series.[2] It was rarer, fortunately, to suffer all three types of abuse in childhood: only 4 per cent of the Representative group of women had such grossly deprived childhoods.

MULTIPLE ABUSE AND DEPRESSION

In the Representative series the experience of at least one of these three abuses was associated with a 34 per cent rate of depression which compared with 11 per cent among women with none of the three abuses – a threefold increase in risk. In the Sisters series similar rates of depression held, at 33 per cent and 14 per cent, respectively. The experience of more than one type of abuse related to an even greater risk of depression. In the Representative series this was most marked for those with all three forms of maltreatment, where over half were depressed in the year before interview. There was little difference between those with one or two abuses, where around 30 per cent rate were depressed. Similar figures held in the Sisters series with a rate of 47 per cent depression among those suffering all three forms of maltreatment, but here there was a clearer gradient with 38 per cent of those with two types of abuse becoming depressed, 26 per cent with one and 14 per cent with none.[3]

FAMILY DIFFICULTIES AND ABUSE

Having established that the more types of abuse a person suffered in childhood the higher the likelihood of depression, we examined whether the presence of other family difficulties similarly increased risk. In the case history given earlier, we saw how neglect and abuse flourished in a web of inter-related family problems, including loss of parent, parental separation and divorce, institutional care, parental discord, parental psychiatric disorder and financial hardship. Such a catalogue of difficulties could serve to increase risk of depression in two ways. First, family difficulties might increase the risk of neglect and abuse which in turn increases risk of depression. Second, such contexts may independently increase risk of later depression. We therefore examined four difficult family contexts to assess the extent to which they were associated with abusive experience and whether they added to the prediction of depression in adult life. The family factors selected were those of parental loss, family discord, poverty and parental psychiatric disorder.

Parental loss

Concerns about the effects of maternal deprivation were first raised in relation to children evacuated away from their families during the Second World War. During the 1950s and 1960s investigators such as John Bowlby and Michael Rutter continued the investigation of this theme in relation to maternal deprivation and separation arising in the context of extended daycare or institutional settings for children. The topic has received additional attention more recently due to interest in the effects of family breakdown as rates of divorce and marital separation continue to increase.

We found loss of mother, defined as death or separation for one continuous year or more before age seventeen, to be highly related to the presence of neglect or abuse. In the Representative London Women series, over half of those with loss of mother suffered neglect or abuse compared with 20 per cent of other women.[4] For multiple abuse the figures were 27 per cent and 7 per cent respectively. As described in earlier chapters, loss of mother was also associated with a doubling of the rate of depression (28 per cent versus 14 per cent). However, in the *absence* of neglect/abuse there was no effect from loss of mother. Some 15 per cent with such a loss but no neglect/abuse became depressed compared with 10 per cent among those with neither factor. It was neglect or abuse which increased the risk of adult disorder rather than the loss itself.[5]

Parental conflict

Parental conflict has been identified in many studies as a risk factor for adult disorder.[6] It is argued that witnessing hostility between parents is so damaging for children that parental separation is often considered preferable to continued parental discord for the children's well-being. Such conflict can vary in degree from poor communication to open arguments or physical violence between parents, as witnessed by the children. For the purposes of our research, we took parental conflict to include open hostility, arguments or violence, rather than milder displays of irritation or tension.

To convey something of the nature of such conflict, the following example describes one woman's experience of growing up in a household dominated by extreme hostility between her parents: 'Dad was always critical of mum. My mum wasn't allowed to read or knit in the living room in front of the TV because my dad didn't like the clicking of the needles or turning the pages. My parents were never affectionate with each other, they argued a lot. It was very, very frightening. Mostly the rows would be over me and my sister. They'd be screaming and shouting, him always saying my mum favoured my sister and mum always saying dad favoured me. They argued over money too and about my father having affairs. They also argued about visitors. My dad didn't like visitors, especially my mum's family. If they came he would sit in the kitchen. The arguments became violent. He'd kick her or punch her in her back, so that the bruises and things didn't show. He never marked her face. I remember one time when I actually thought he was going to kill her. He tried to strangle her, he was out of his senses. More and more as I got older they'd smash things. He threw a whole bowl of washing up at mum. He'd throw his dinner at her if he was in a bad mood.' This example features severe parental hostility which formed a backdrop to the antipathy and physical abuse experienced by the child. Her father regularly beat her with a cane or a belt, or his fists: 'Once I got thrown across the room and got my mouth split open on the wooden part of the settee when I was about eight. I was frightened as a child.'

Hostility between parents was highly associated with the experience of neglect or abuse in childhood in our Sisters series, with as many as 71 per cent of children in conflictful families suffering at least one abuse compared with 29 per cent of those in homes which did not feature parental conflict.[7] When multiple abuses were examined the relationship between neglect/abuse and parental conflict was even greater. Some 40 per cent of women raised in conflictful homes experienced multiple abuse compared with 9 per cent of those raised in more peaceable contexts. When depression was examined in relation to both conflict and neglect/abuse, again only the *latter* showed a significant relationship. There was no relationship between parental conflict and depression, with 27 per cent from discordant households becoming depressed versus 22 per cent from households without conflict. Again, it was neglect or abuse which was responsible for more than doubling the rate of depression.[8]

Poverty

Neglect of children is often linked with poverty, conjuring up images from Victorian times of children lacking food, clothing, hygiene and education. Although neglect often did occur alongside poverty, the links between the two were complex. For example, we encountered neglect arising in materially adequate circumstances and even in situations of comparative wealth. In some instances finances were sufficient but poverty was imposed on the child, as in the following example: 'My father always had a good job, but he used money for power so he would keep my mother extremely short of money and would also make her beg for her housekeeping money. He wouldn't give it to her till 4.30 on a Saturday, just before the shops shut, so she'd have to be crying before she got it. There was no money spent on us. As a teenager I had to have boys' clothes that could be passed on to my brother, in the interest of economy. He kept my mother short of money so she was restricted in the choice of food she could buy. On a personal level there wasn't a share-out of wealth. Father would either ignore birthdays or he might get me something that he knew I didn't want, or give me something that was needed for the house, say it was mine and then put restrictions on using it.'

Where financial deprivation does occur, it is often assumed to give rise to neglect of children, and subsequent adult disorder. Yet many examples can be cited of individuals rising from poor origins to become stable, fully functioning adults. If the association between poverty and neglect was strong, children brought up during economic depressions such as that of the 1930s would be assumed to have equally suffered from neglect. However, historical material and biographies show this was not uniformly the case.[9] In fact current popular opinion at times adopts the reverse position and sees affluence and associated commercialism as a barrier to good childcare, with children exposed to new types of hazards involving uncontrolled television viewing, access to designer-labelled clothes, drugs and alcohol. Recent work shows how *increases* in disorders of childhood in the post-war period have occurred at a time when poverty in the Western world has *decreased*.[10]

Nevertheless, it is also true that a shortage of financial resources can lead to stressors on families which affect the children. For example, lack of money can often be a source of tension and conflict between parents. Difficulties such as long-term unemployment and mounting debts can contribute to parental psychiatric disorder too. Conversely, financial difficulty may follow from parents spending on alcohol or gambling. Lack of resources may lead to both parents having to work unusually long hours outside the home, resulting in some cases to neglect of children. Poverty may compound other risk factors: following the loss of one parent the remaining parent may face the financial burden of providing for the children single-handedly.

To investigate the role of poverty, we asked the women who participated in our Sisters series about material hardship experienced during their childhood, including the presence of financial or housing difficulties, or extended periods of parental unemployment. Like parental conflict, poverty was highly related to the presence of neglect or abuse, with double the rate among women with material hardship (77 per cent versus 38 per cent). For multiple abuse the association was more striking with a three-fold increase: 45 per cent of those in poor homes had more than one abuse compared with 15 per cent with no poverty.[11] However, there was no association of childhood poverty with adult depression, with 29 per cent from poor families becoming depressed compared with 22 per cent from more affluent households. Again, neglect or abuse alone was responsible for increase in depressive risk.[12]

Parental psychiatric state

Parental psychiatric disorder has long been used as a risk marker for disorder in the children. The rationale for such a link encompasses both genetic explanations, whereby children are argued to inherit genes for a particular disorder from their parents, and environmental explanations whereby parents' psychiatric disorder impedes their competent parenting.[13, 14] More subtle environmental links have also been suggested whereby parents' psychiatric disorder results from their own early experience of poor parenting which they repeat on their own children. The following analysis only concerns the possible added *environmental* risks for the offspring of parents with psychiatric problems. Unfortunately, our study design did not allow for the investigation of possible genetic effects.

To assess parental psychiatric disorder we asked women for their recollections of their parents' emotional and behavioural problems, present when the women themselves were growing up. The disorder we focused on was primarily that of alcohol abuse defined in terms of problem drinking. We chose this disorder because it was one of the most readily observable by the children in the household, and various studies have linked this with depression in daughters.[15]

In the selected Sisters series we found no higher rate of neglect or abuse in general for women with an alcoholic parent. However, *multiple* abuse was almost twice as common in such households (40 per cent versus 24 per cent with no alcoholic parent).[16] Alcoholism of parents was unrelated to later depression in the women, with 27 per cent of those with an alcoholic parent becoming depressed in adult life compared with 24 per cent with no such parental disorder. When examined together it was clear that neglect and abuse alone raised risk of depression.[17]

PARENTS' COPING WITH FAMILY DIFFICULTIES

So far we have seen that loss of a parent, parental conflict, parental alcohol abuse and family poverty are associated with maltreatment of children. While these family problems occur more commonly with abuse of children, the latter is by no means a necessary consequence. Among the many hundreds of childhood histories collected, we were struck by examples of parents' efforts to provide a secure, safe and loving home for their children despite adverse personal circumstances such as financial hardship and marital breakdown.

To convey the efforts of some parents, here is one woman's experience of being raised in a single-parent household following the death of her father. Though short of money, her mother ensured that the children were never neglected: 'We couldn't have things that we'd seen other children having. Mother would say "We haven't got that sort of money." She did really well with what money she did have. A lot of our clothes came from jumble sales. It was always good stuff, and if it wasn't she'd make it good. We had bread and jam for tea, unlike my friends who had cooked meals. Life was very difficult for mum. Money was tight, she had two jobs, one so that she could be there when we came back from school, and then once we were in bed, a neighbour used to look after us while she went out again to an usherette's job. She'd buy hand-knitted jumpers at jumble sales and unpick them and reknit them. Where she got the time for that I don't know.' This particular woman did not experience depression in adult life.

Another woman recounted how well she was cared for in

childhood by her mother despite the fact that her father drank and her parent's marriage suffered as a result: 'Mother was quite strict, but a calm, fair person, she took things very reasonably. She never hit us. We were well looked after. I think she used to try to laugh off the problems with my father, but she was very quiet in those days, quite subdued sometimes. I don't remember father looking after us very much. He didn't participate really.' After her parents separated, the children remained with mother: 'Some of my happiest memories are after the divorce with just my mother and the children at home. My mother certainly looked a lot healthier. I really enjoyed that time. I certainly was much happier.'

A similar account can be found in descriptions of poor families in Victorian London. Consider Mayhew's account of a girl street seller who describes poverty but not neglect: 'There's six on us in family and father and mother that makes eight. Father used to do odd jobs with the gas pipes in the streets, and when work was slack we had very hard times of it. Mother always liked being with us at home, and used to manage to keep us employed and out of mischief . . . . She's been very good to us has mother, and so's father. She always liked to hear us reading to her while she was washing or such like! . . . If I've done well [selling apples] she'll say "come you're a good hand at it; you've done famous". Yes mother's very fair that way. . . . My parents is very fair to me.'[18]

In households such as these, resilience and resourcefulness of parents resulted in children being protected from suffering, even if the family problems themselves could not be resolved. In the short term the children avoided neglect and abuse, and in the long term this led to a reduction in their child's risk of depression.

EARLY CAUSES OF DEPRESSION

It can be seen that some early experiences are more critically damaging than others. Pin-pointing the most important of these various factors is a complex task, especially when one considers that in human experience unpleasant or stressful events rarely crop up in isolation. Most develop in the context of a sequence of accumulating difficulty. Consider for instance the stressful childhood experience of parental separation and divorce. This may be preceded by periods of conflict between parents and followed by financial hardship and further conflict surrounding custody and access to the children. Once responsibility for the children passes to step-parents or other adults, new conflicts can arise and neglect and abuse are then more likely to occur. Thus even an apparently circumscribed childhood experience such as separation from a parent can occur in a stream of related risk factors. Being able to identify the key component denoting risk for later disorder in the children in such a sequence of related crises is part of the measurement task in social science research.

Scientific investigation is required, not only to establish an association between one factor and another, but in order to develop theories and models whereby one factor is identified as the *cause* of another. Thus whether the first factor in some way produces the second and the link between the two can be seen as part of the same underlying process. Therefore if neglect/abuse in childhood was a cause of depression it would need to be shown to be part of the process by which depression occurs and alternative causes eliminated. The standard method of testing for causal links in laboratory experimental studies has been expressed in the following metaphor as: 'The operation of "waggling" one variable in order to determine if it causes some other variable to "move", and doing so in such a way as to find out if this "movement" is brought about systematically and regularly in varying circumstances.'[19]

Applying this principle to the study of psychosocial risk for depressive disorder is difficult. The 'waggling' of antecedent conditions systematically in naturalistic settings such as those described in this book, is difficult if not impossible to perform. Since we wanted to examine whether the initial association found between neglect/abuse in childhood and depression in adulthood represented a real causal connection between the two, all we could do was to see if when the first varied in some way, the second could be seen to be similarly affected.

Two ways of testing whether one factor causes another have already been shown in this chapter. The first concerns evidence of what is known as a 'dose–response' relationship between two factors. If there is a true causal connection then the higher the 'dosage' of neglect and abuse experienced in childhood, the higher the 'response' expected in terms of later adult depression. As already described, we did find evidence of this, with the greater the number of abuses experienced in childhood the higher the rate of depression experienced in later life. A second means of checking whether one factor causes another is to examine whether the apparent association could actually be due to some third factor related to both. We have considered in this chapter four other factors which *may* have provided better links with depression than neglect or abuse. However, the analysis has shown that each of these failed to relate to depression in the absence of neglect or abuse. Thus we can begin to assume that neglect/abuse in childhood is at least one of the causes of adult depression.

The relationship between family context and child neglect/abuse is of great interest in itself, and gives some clues as to the way in which child maltreatment arises. Each of the family context factors studied proved to be not only associated with the presence of neglect or abuse, but to increase with an increase of abuse. This new 'dose–response' effect again suggests a causal linkage and although we cannot be completely sure of the exact temporal order (for example whether abuse follows parental conflict or vice versa), the family context factors may prove to represent an earlier causal link in the chain from neglect/abuse to depression. The exploration of such factors allows us to consider how and why abuse occurs, and to identify families which may be at risk for such maltreatment of children.

IMPLICATIONS FOR SOCIAL POLICY

The importance of unearthing the causal links between childhood experience and adult depression cannot be stressed too highly. Social policy requires reliable evidence upon which to build appropriate strategies for prevention and intervention. At times, however, contradictory action is implied. If, for example, separation from a parent is deemed to be the true earlier cause of adult depression then policy implications would advocate that we reduce its prevalence and direct resources towards cementing family relations. If, in contrast, parental discord preceding parental separation rather than the parental separation *per se* is identified as the main risk, then an opposing policy may be advocated, namely that marital break-up could be beneficial where it protects a child from being further damaged by prolonged conflict between parents. A number of studies in the late 1970s and early 1980s variously showed parental loss or marital discord to increase risk of disorder in adult life. If not further explored, this anomaly could lead to contradictory recommendations for policy-makers and professionals involved in the care and treatment of children. In fact we have shown in our series that greater damage emanates from neglect or abuse of children than either loss or discord. This illustrates the value in continuing to search for critical risk factors and those closer to the mechanisms by which damage occurs.

These findings have implications for family intervention aimed at reducing a child's chances of developing depression. Such intervention could take many different forms and each solution represents a costly decision, not only in monetary terms but also in terms of the human misery involved for the family members if the solution fails. Choosing the most effective intervention relies first on knowing which factors give rise to abuse and neglect, and second which factors are critical for increasing risk of later depression. During the course of our research we encountered many women brought up in the adversity 'cocktail' of abuse and neglect in combination with family difficulties. Using their experiences we were able to explore the role of the various problems operating in circumstances such as this, to understand their relationship both to each other and to depression.

CONCLUSION

From an analysis of childhood maltreatment in conjunction with a number of family characteristics, it has been possible to begin to understand the origins of child abuse. These associations are important in that they give some clue to the nature of the social and material environment in which abuse occurs. Drawing all the strands of the analysis together, a picture emerges of maltreatment arising in families under a great deal of stress. Typically, in such families the parent's marriage is either seriously disintegrating or has actually broken down in the midst of difficulties such as unemployment, mounting debt or inadequate housing. Some turn to alcohol as a means of coping, which further compounds the problem. While this tangled web of disadvantage needs further exploration, it is safe to say that such challenging circumstances at times affect parents' ability to raise their children. The ultimate victims of such adversity are, of course, the children themselves. However, when these adverse family circumstances are present but neglect or abuse absent, there are no long-term harmful effects on the children insofar as raised risk of adult depression is concerned. Thus it would appear that individuals can rise above poverty, parental loss and their parents' poor marriages to become fully functioning adults.

NOTES

1 Caprara, V. and Rutter, M. (1995) 'Individual development and social change', in Rutter, M. and Smith, D. (eds) *Psychosocial Disorders in Young People. Time Trends and their Causes*, Chichester, UK: Wiley and Sons.

2 In the Representative London Women series 29% (82/286) of the total group experienced at least one of: neglect, physical or sexual abuse at a 'marked' or 'moderate' level and 12% (34/286) had multiple abuse in terms of *two* or more. Only 4% (11/286) suffered all three experiences of neglect, physical *and* sexual abuse before age seventeen.

3 *Table 8.1* Multiple abuse – neglect, physical abuse or sexual abuse – and depression (% depressed)

Neglect/abuse	Representative London Women series	Sisters series
3 factors	55 (6/11) ⎫	47 (7/15) ⎫
2 factors	30 (7/23) ⎬ 34%	38 (15/40) ⎬ 33%
1 factor	31 (15/48) ⎭	26 (14/53) ⎭
None	11 (22/204)	14 (13/90)
	p < 0.001	p < 0.005

4 In the Representative London Women series 54% (40/74) of those with loss of mother under seventeen had experienced either neglect or abuse compared with 20% (42/212) of women with no loss of mother (p < 0.001). Multiple neglect or abuse occurred for 27% (20/74) of those with maternal loss compared with 7% (14/212) of remaining women (p < 0.001). Loss of mother was defined as death or separation for 12 months continuously before age seventeen.

5 *Table 8.2* Loss of mother and neglect/abuse (Representative London Women series)

Neglect/abuse	Loss of mother		
	Loss	No loss	
Present	40 (16/40)	29 (12/42)	NS
Absent	15 (5/34)	10 (17/170)	NS
Total	28 (21/74)	14 (29/212)	p < 0.01

6 Jenkins, J.M. and Smith, M.A. (1991) 'Marital disharmony and children's behaviour problems. Aspects of a poor marriage that affect children adversely', *Journal of Child Psychology and Psychiatry 32*: 793–810.

7 In the Sisters series 71% (85/120) of those with parental conflict experienced neglect or abuse compared with 29% (23/78) of those with no parental conflict (p < 0.001). In terms of multiple abuse the

figures were 40% (48/120) compared with 9% (7/78) respectively (p < 0.001). Parental conflict was defined as either marked discord, high antipathy between parents or violence between parents before the child was seventeen.

8 *Table 8.3* Parental conflict, neglect/abuse and depression (Sisters series) (% depressed)

Neglect/abuse	Parental conflict		
	Present	Absent	
Present	34 (29/85)	30 (7/23)	NS
Absent	9 (3/35)	18 (10/55)	NS
Total	27 (32/120)	22 (17/78)	NS

9 Elder, G. (1974) *Children of the Great Depression*, Chicago and London: University of Chicago Press.

10 Rutter, M. and Smith, D. (eds) (1995) *Psychosocial Disorders in Young People. Time Trends and their Causes*, Chichester, UK: Wiley and Sons.

11 In the Sisters series 77% (65/84) of those with family poverty experienced either neglect or abuse compared with 38% (43/114) with no family poverty (p < 0.001). The figures for multiple abuse were 45% (38/84) compared with 15% (17/114) respectively (p < 0.001). Family poverty was defined in terms of either severe housing problems, financial difficulty or father's unemployment before the child was seventeen.

12 *Table 8.4* Family poverty, neglect/abuse and depression (Sisters series) (% depressed)

Neglect/abuse	Family poverty		
	Present	Absent	
Present	32 (21/65)	35 (15/43)	NS
Absent	16 (3/19)	14 (10/71)	NS
Total	29 (24/84)	22 (25/114)	NS

13 Hammen, C. (1991) *Depression Runs in Families. The Social Context of Risk and Resilience in Children of Depressed Mothers*, New York: Springer-Verlag.

14 Plommin, R. (1996) 'Beyond nature versus nurture', in Hall, Laura Lee (ed.) *Genetics and Mental Illness. Evolving Issues for Research and Society*, New York, London: Plenum Press,

15 Kendler, K., Heath, A., Neale, M., Kessler, R. and Eaves, L. (1993) 'Alcoholism and major depression in women: a twin study of the causes of comorbidity', *Archives General Psychiatry 50*: 690–698.

16 In the Sisters series, among those with a parent with alcohol problems 63% (30/48) experienced neglect or abuse, compared with 52%

(78/150) of those with no alcoholic parent (NS). For multiple abuse the figures are 40% (19/48) and 24% (36/150) respectively (p < 0.10).

17   *Table 8.5* Parental alcohol problems, neglect/abuse and depression (Sisters series) (% depressed)

Neglect/abuse	Parental alcohol problems		
	Present	Absent	
Present	37 (11/30)	32 (25/78)	NS
Absent	11 (2/18)	15 (11/72)	NS
Total	27 (13/48)	24 (36/150)	NS

18   Mayhew, H. (1851: 93) *Mayhew's London*, London: Spring Books.
19   Rutter and Smith (1995: 7) op. cit. note 10.

Chapter 9

Adult vulnerability: legacy of childhood

A child who has a history of abuse expects others to be rejecting, hostile, and unavailable. A child who has been neglected (physically, emotionally, or both) expects others to be unresponsive, unavailable, and not willing to meet his or her needs. Maltreated children bring these expectations to relationships, and they respond to others in a fashion consistent with their expectations.

(Egeland 1993: 206)[1]

In order to understand how adverse experiences in early life can make an impact some twenty or thirty years later, our interviews have documented the life histories of women stretching from childhood to mid-adulthood. From their biographical details we have been able to map out sequences of influential events, and search for patterns of experience held in common among vulnerable women. It is evident from childhood accounts that abused children frequently enter adulthood in a vulnerable condition, with a damaged view of self and others, compounded by poor coping skills. For some women, such childhood vulnerability sets them along a pathway of further damaging experiences resulting in clinical depression in adult life. It is this accumulation of risk across the lifespan rather than a single negative occurrence which has proved particularly detrimental to later mental health.

To illustrate the chain of experiences which can lead from childhood maltreatment to adult vulnerability and consequent depression, we begin by recounting the life histories of two women who were typical of many that took part in our research. While on the surface the two women appeared to have very different and contrasting life experience, they nevertheless shared certain features which are characteristic of many women who are neglected or abused as children. First, both possessed a damaged self-image. Their failure to form close bonds with parents in childhood combined with a lack of love and care in early years had created deficiencies in their view of themselves as worthy or lovable, and effective copers. These negative feelings were compounded by family members in childhood. The second feature these women shared was a damaged view of human relationships. Early experience had taught them to expect little from others, since those they had loved and trusted had hurt them most. The third feature they shared was the experience of entrapment in punishing situations and relationships, with few alternative rewarding roles. The first woman, a thirty-year-old insurance clerk, was single and childless, working full-time and living at home with her parents when we interviewed her. The second woman, a forty-year-old foster mother, was in her second marriage with five children and had additional charge of two foster children.

THE INSURANCE CLERK'S EARLY LIFE

The insurance clerk was one of five children brought up in poor surroundings by neglectful and inattentive parents. Her mother was a moody and irritable woman who physically abused her in childhood. Her father, with whom she had little contact, was emotionally distant. Her elder brother sexually abused her over a number of years and forced her to remain silent about the abuse. Her school life was marred by teasing and bullying, including taunting from teachers. She had no close relationships or support figures in her early life.

She experienced a lack of opportunity and personal growth in later life, hampered by her helplessness and timidity. She left school at sixteen to start work in her present office. She had continued in the same job for fourteen years without advancement or promotion, developing no social life or friendships with colleagues. She met her only boyfriend when she was twenty-five but the relationship lasted only six months. She described the relationship as being one-sided: 'I liked him, he was a nice chap. I was attracted to him, but I think he liked me more than I liked him. I felt distant. I was a bit shy and I think I was afraid of getting too close really. I couldn't really talk to him. We broke up when I said I couldn't marry him. He kept coming round but eventually he got the message that I wasn't that interested.' She had made no subsequent relationships with men, and avoided situations where there might be opportunities to develop intimate ties. When we interviewed her she was socially isolated, without any fulfilling role in her life.

THE FOSTER MOTHER'S EARLY LIFE

The second woman lost her mother as a baby and was brought up by her father. In childhood she experienced antipathy from her father who was more critical of her more than of her siblings, particularly when she was the only one who failed to get into grammar school. He forced her to do much of the housework while never requiring her brothers to help. He was also physically abusive to her. When she was fourteen she had a particularly unpleasant row with her father in which he told her with some satisfaction that her mother was not really dead, but a 'whore' who had abandoned her and the other children. He accused her of being like her mother.

At the age of sixteen she had an unplanned pregnancy with a young man she had only known a few months. On hearing the news her father knocked her across the room with a blow to the face, then threw her out of the house. She tried to abort the pregnancy with the help of a friend but failed. Having nowhere else to go, she moved in with her boyfriend whom she then married. The marriage was difficult from the beginning, as her new husband proved to be controlling and possessive. She was unable to work because of child-care responsibilities, and her partner kept her short of money, hardly giving her enough for household expenses. He wouldn't let her see friends or go out to work even when the first child was at school. They both wanted a large family and she had five children in the first ten years of marriage. Her husband wanted even more children. Thus at the age of twenty-seven she was trapped in an unsupportive and restricting marriage with five children, the eldest of whom was ten years old, the youngest a baby. The relationship continued to deteriorate and eventually ended when the youngest child was five. After some years alone she married a man recovering from alcohol dependence, and took on two stepchildren from his previous marriage. When we interviewed her she was having problems in this second marriage, as her husband had turned again to alcohol.

THE TWO WOMEN'S ADULT LIVES

While these women clearly found themselves in very different circumstances, both had poor support at the time we saw them.

The insurance clerk had become isolated and lonely. Although living with her parents and younger sister, she had no closeness to her family. There was conflict in the relationship with her mother which had been present since childhood: 'I still feel a lot of resentment towards her. I do feel close in a sense, but I can't really tell her. She's moody and difficult to get on with. She's not at all happy about the idea I might move out.' She was somewhat closer to her father although felt unable to show it: 'I have a lot of respect for him, he's more intelligent than my mum. If I wanted any sensible advice I'd go to my dad rather than my mum.' However, she confided little and the relationship lacked warmth. She was on friendly but distant terms with her siblings, but with her older abusive brother she refused any contact at all.

Her life was devoid of any close relationships: 'I can't trust, that's the bottom line of it really. If you talk to someone at work, you always feel its going to get back to someone else, because that's how they are. I've had two good friends since I left school. My really best friend lives abroad now and another lives outside London. So I don't get to see them anymore.' She reported wanting a close relationship but this was blocked by fears about revealing her feelings. She found the company of others boring or irritating and she was unable to relax in social situations.

The foster mother was surrounded by a large family but paradoxically had no-one to support her emotionally. The relationship with her second husband had been difficult for about eighteen months before we saw her. She couldn't confide her problems in him, finding him critical and judgemental. He was unreliable and careless with money, resulting in financial difficulties for the family. They had recently had a serious row, after which she left for the night, saying she was leaving him permanently. However, she returned and he forbade her to leave again. In arguments he was verbally abusive and aggressive, pushing her and ripping her blouse on one occasion. She found him frightening, particularly when he was drunk. She frequently apologised for things which she knew were not her fault, just to keep the peace.

Despite these problems, she reported feeling very dependent on her husband, and being unable to cope when apart from him: 'When my husband is away its horrible. He was working away for about nine weeks earlier this year, and he was coming home weekends, but the last few weeks he had to stay there to get the job finished and that was hell.' She described how much she loved him, but wasn't sure that he would always be there when she needed him.

She reported feeling emotionally close to her large family and described close links with her adult son, talking to him on the phone a few times every day. She felt a need for frequent contact: 'It doesn't bother me if I haven't got friends, as long as I have my family.' Despite close contact with her son, she felt unable to lean on him at times of crises. Indeed, she was unable to identify even one person in whom she could confide fully and who would provide her with emotional support. She felt suspicious of people outside the family: 'I'm not very trusting. I suppose it's because I've done things for people and they've turned round and been ungrateful.'

Both the insurance clerk and the foster mother had low self-esteem when we saw them. The insurance clerk described herself in these terms: 'I'm a bit shy, a bit of a loner at times. I'm very good at hiding my feelings. I can seem happy-go-lucky, walk around as if I haven't a care in the world, but it just isn't me.' She had recently been thinking about her childhood experience of sexual abuse and linked many of her negative feelings about herself to that time: 'Sometimes I just hate myself, I blame myself for having let the abuse happen.' She had experienced similar feelings in childhood, suggesting her poor self-esteem was a long-term characteristic: 'I felt my sister was better at everything than I was. I felt I wasn't good enough, I never felt as good as her. I felt worthless and had difficulty coming to terms with what had happened to me.'

When asked about positive aspects of herself she replied: 'I don't think I have any good qualities. My worst feature is that I'm very aggressive at times. I'm also too sympathetic at times. I'm just the sort of person who finds it hard to say "no" if somebody needs something. I do things just to please people, to get them to like me. That's my weakness.' When asked about her feelings of competence in her different roles she felt she was poor at social relationships: 'As far as my personal life is concerned I back off from people too much. People just walk all over me, which has happened many times. People include me in social evenings and I can't say no. I try to put on a brave face but I'm not enjoying myself, I just don't want to be bad-mannered.' The only areas in which she felt she functioned well were at work and in caring for her parents.

There were similarities with the foster mother's view of herself. When asked to describe herself she said: 'I can be very sympathetic but also very hard. I've had to be because of the way I was brought up. In this day and age you've got to be hard. But I will give anything to anybody. My brother came to live with me when he had nowhere to go and I was happy to help. But then he took advantage. If you do too much for people they dump on you. That's my problem, I do too much for others. I never put myself first. I put the kids first. It's bad, I give them too much.'

She had negative feelings about herself in other areas too: 'I feel people are looking at me because I'm overweight and thinking, "Look at that fat bitch." It's the main thing about myself that I want to change. I'm also very quick-tempered and very moody. I'm a very sensitive person, I get very emotional. I'm not happy but I will put on a cheerful face to the world, even though I get very low. I get angry at people sometimes and people think I'm wicked and evil but it's something I can't help.' When asked about positive characteristics, she reported some good feelings about herself in her different roles: 'I think I am a good wife, I do a lot more than other people. Very few women do what I do. I am a good mum. I think I love the kids too much sometimes. I'd give my children anything.'

HISTORY OF DEPRESSION

Both of these women had suffered more than one depressive episode in their lives. The insurance clerk had her first episode at age fifteen when she tried to commit suicide because of the torment of her childhood years. She became depressed again after the relationship with her boyfriend ended. The depression lasted for nearly a year but she sought no treatment. Her third and current episode of depression began just over a year before she was interviewed, when her father became an invalid after a heart operation resulting in his need for constant care. Since her mother was also in ill-health, both parents became reliant on her. Prior to this she had been making plans to leave home but, following her father's illness, she began to feel trapped with no possibility of leading a life of her own.

The unrewarding situation she found herself in provoked a clinical depression which was present when we saw her: 'Most of the day I'm walking about in a daydream. My mind goes blank and I have trouble concentrating at work. I go to work, come home, have my dinner and go upstairs and no-one sees me again until the next morning. I don't feel like eating any more and I've let my appearance go. My bedroom doesn't get tidied or cleaned for weeks on end. I feel that nothing is worth the effort. The future is very bleak, I just feel there is no way out. I don't see myself as ever changing. Everything is too much effort. It's not worth it. Just living seems too much of an effort. I feel I just don't want to be here this time next week.' She felt suicidal three months before interview and telephoned the Samaritans helpline. For the first time she had disclosed the sexual abuse she was subjected to in childhood. She refused the offer of seeing a Samaritans counsellor but nevertheless felt an enormous sense of relief after finally telling someone about her abusive early life.

The foster mother experienced her initial episode of depression when her first marriage broke up in her late twenties. She lost weight and couldn't sleep or concentrate. She felt hopeless about her situation, but never considered taking her own life because of her children. She avoided seeing others: 'For the first six months after he left I didn't go out at all, but at least I knew I could if I wanted to. There was no one to stop me this time.' Eventually she began to recover and started going out. For the first time in her life she was unhindered by either an overbearing father or controlling partner: 'I spent two years on my own with the five children. It was great. I was able to go out with my friend and start enjoying life. I was living on benefit when we first split up, but I couldn't stand it so I went and got a job. I worked full-time in a shop.'

She became depressed again in the year we saw her due to a deterioration in her second marriage. Her husband's unreliability and drinking worsened following a row he had with his daughter (her stepdaughter). He then had a row with his manager at work which resulted in him being made redundant. This placed even greater financial strain on the family. His drinking increased, and one night led to a violent row with his wife: 'He got paralytically drunk. I thought he was going to kill me. He punched me. He ripped my kitchen to bits. I had to get the police because he scared me. He had been drinking all day and returned in the evening. He just started hitting me. I had bruises all over. I regretted calling the police because they wanted to take him to the police station then and there. I told them not to because he's never done it before. They said if they have another call from me they'll take him and charge him. He's like a split personality when he's drunk. I've seen him nasty before but not that bad. I've told him that if he does it again I'll call the police and have him arrested. I've thought of separating. I do love him, I know it sounds silly. I don't want to leave him but it makes me think its going to happen one day. If he carries on the way he is there's no way I can cope with his drinking. I think I'd cope much better on my own.'

She became depressed soon after this attack: 'I cry quite a lot. I don't think there has been a week gone past when I haven't cried. I feel hopeless about the future, that things will never get better. I don't think things could get worse. Its been absolute hell. There's nothing I can do, is there? I feel life isn't worth living at times.'

SCARS FROM CHILDHOOD

In terms of the lasting impact of early experience, it seems that the insurance clerk had never in effect moved away from her childhood entrapment and her individuality had never been allowed to develop. Without encouragement and help from others she had made few efforts to become independent and improve her life. She had found no opportunity to leave home, get further education or start a family of her own. There had been no reconciliation with her parents despite their increased dependence on her, no recognition of, or reparation for, her sexual abuse, no real achievement in her job, and no friendships outside the home. Her only relationship with a man faltered because of her timidity. Her helplessness was compounded by low self-esteem and fear of others which increased her entrapment. At each new disappointment or setback she slipped from helplessness to hopelessness and ultimately into depression.

The foster mother's adverse adult life was also understandable in terms of her childhood experience. At an early age she became trapped through pregnancy in a loveless marriage and weighed down with mothering responsibilities. Such events might have been avoided had she received help from a mother who could advise her about sexual relationships and contraception. Having heavy responsibilities at an early age impeded her ability to mature and find a suitable partner, build a career and financial security, and embark on motherhood at a time when she felt ready. We can also see how her psychological make-up hindered her efforts at coping with such adversity. Her self-esteem had been chronically poor, and she felt undeserving of love and care. As a consequence she settled for a lower quality of support from her partner than many would – she was grateful that someone loved her regardless of their suitability. She was also impeded by her negative feelings about relationships: her mistrust and anger combined with high dependency would have provided difficulties in any but the most patient of partner relationships. Thus, both the insurance clerk and foster mother, via different routes, found themselves in circumstances which were to render them susceptible to depression in adult life.

Depression is an unsurprising outcome following childhood maltreatment when one considers the minimum requirements for psychological growth and development. Three main clusters of needs have been identified as necessary for psychological health by psychologists such as Abraham Maslow.[2] The first is *safety* and being protected from the dangers of the environment. The second is *support* in terms of the love, respect and a sense of belonging achieved through positive contact with close others. The third is *self-esteem* and a sense of worth arising from being valued by others and experiencing success and achievement in one role or another. All three hinge on the presence of other people with whom one has ongoing close, supportive relationships and a history of intimacy and trust. These needs were clearly unmet in the abusive childhoods discussed in previous chapters. The children were first and foremost unsafe. Not only did parents and those close by fail to protect them, but these same people were often themselves the source of danger. The children received little support, their social world was either bare or hostile, and there was no source of comfort, respect or belonging needed for growth. When a child's basic psychological and physical needs are unmet, the result is a stunting of psychological growth and self-esteem, a failure to thrive, and a deprivation of opportunity extending into adult life.

TEENAGE AND EARLY ADULT VULNERABILITY

Some experiences focused on teenage years were particularly imbued with risk for later life. These included early, unplanned and unsupported pregnancy, as illustrated by the case history of the foster mother. We found that in our Loss of Mother series, 35 per cent of women with an early maternal loss who were neglected in childhood later experienced an unplanned pregnancy while not living with a partner compared with 7 per cent of those without neglect. An unplanned and unsupported pregnancy was also related to an increased risk of depression in later life: 42 per cent with such a pregnancy became depressed in the year before interview compared with 15 per cent of other women.[3] Pregnancy in these conditions also related to lower support from a partner in *later* adult life which also carried risk for depression.[4]

One of the consequences of early and unplanned parenthood was a period of time spent as a single parent. This arose either as a direct consequence of the unplanned pregnancy or later, when the first relationship failed, as in the foster mother's life. Contrary to popular belief, single parenthood is usually a temporary situation, and is more commonly the result of a relationship breakdown rather than never having lived with the father of the child. Single mothers had double the rate of depression of married or cohabiting mothers (16 per cent versus 8 per cent), and much of this depression could be traced back to the break-up of the previous relationship.[5]

For some women the abuse received in childhood was echoed in early adult life. As we have seen in the case of the foster mother, childhood neglect and physical abuse from a domineering parent can be substituted in later life for physical attacks from a violent partner. Sexual assaults in adult life were also fairly common though not exclusively from partner. In our Representative London Women series, 27 per cent of women had experienced violence or sexual assault from a partner or similar assault from another male in adulthood.[6] This proportion is chillingly similar to the rate of child-hood neglect or abuse in the same series. The presence of physical or sexual assaults in early adult life was highly related to childhood neglect or abuse: 44 per cent of those with childhood neglect or abuse had suffered *adult* physical or sexual abuse as compared with 21 per cent of the remaining women.[7] Such abuse in adulthood related to later episodes of disorder: almost a third of those who had experienced earlier adult abuse were depressed in the year we saw them compared with 13 per cent of remaining women.[8] These proportions mirror those found in the analysis of childhood mal-treatment.

The combination of maltreatment both in childhood *and* in adult life presents a potent risk for depression. Some 42 per cent of those with *both* of these types of experiences became depressed in the year of interview, a rate almost double that seen among those who experienced one alone (25 per cent). This compares with a rate of only 8 per cent among those who experienced neither.[9] Not only was depression more common among women with both childhood and adulthood abusive experiences, but such women were also more likely to suffer chronic, more debilitating episodes of depression, lasting a year or longer.[10] We heard one particularly unfortunate story of a teenage pregnancy resulting from a sexual assault. The woman involved had experienced a neglectful and physically abusive childhood. She was then violently raped when aged nineteen by a boyfriend she had known only briefly. She became pregnant and kept the baby, unsupported by family or friends over a number of years. In adult life she experienced chronically low self-esteem and loneliness, accompanied by periodic bouts of depression.

LATER ADULT VULNERABILITY

The circumstances known to immediately precede an episode of clinical depression in adult life have been closely studied by our research team over many years. Results show that the critical factors which render a woman vulnerable to an imminent episode of depression are low self-esteem and difficulties in relationships entailing poor support. To assess low self-esteem, negative comments about the self were taken into account. Relevant material included comments concerning personal attributes such as appearance, personality, intelligence and ability, as well as feelings of inadequacy and failure in roles such as parenthood, or as a partner, worker or home-maker. Often the comments were highly rejecting of the self and demonstrated a sense of worthlessness and inferiority as illustrated in the two case histories described earlier.

Such low self-esteem proved to be highly related to the second vulnerability factor predicting depression, namely difficulties in relationships. For married or cohabiting women, this included an unsupportive relationship with partner characterised by low confiding and a high degree of conflict. For women without a partner, poor support involved the lack of a close confidant. As expected, neglect and abuse in childhood were highly related to these adult vulnerability factors: of those with childhood neglect or abuse as many as 71 per cent of women had low self-esteem or poor support in adulthood compared with 48 per cent of those without such childhood maltreatment.[11]

LIFE CRISES

In adulthood, depression itself is typically activated by a severe life crisis, such as the break-up of a marriage or the loss of a job. When faced with such severely unpleasant events, particularly those involving relationships, vulnerable women are very likely to become depressed. Vulnerability could be seen as the psychological equiva-lent to deficiency in the immune system, not in itself causing illness but making the individual prey to any 'viral infections' present in the environment.[12] When attacked by the 'viruses' of life crises the individual with depleted inner resources succumbs to hopelessness, self-loathing and depression.

Such crises were common in the inner-city areas we studied: half the working-class women of the Representative London sample experienced at least one in a twelve-month period. However, only a fifth of women became depressed following such a crisis and these proved to be women with prior adult vulnerability. The adult vulner-ability factors were also highly prevalent: half of the Representative sample had either poor support or low self-esteem when interviewed, and a quarter had both of these factors simultaneously. However, what proved to be rare was the juxtaposition of all three experiences in time: the combination of poor support, low self-esteem and a life crisis. Among the Representative sample, only one in twenty experi-enced such a combination in any one year, yet the combination of all three factors had devastating consequences: 46 per cent (22/48) became depressed within twelve months compared with 4 per cent (10/255) of all women without this adverse combination.[13, 14]

CHANGES IN VULNERABILITY

Our results suggest that depression may occur at any time of life that a woman finds herself plagued by feelings of inadequacy, accom-panied by a lack of support from her partner or close friends, and facing a serious life crisis. In this sense vulnerability to depression is both a characteristic of an *individual*, indicated by psychological factors such as low self-esteem, mistrust and fear of others, as well as a characteristic of a *situation*, involving high rates of life events and involvement with unreliable and hostile others. However, it is important to realise that a woman's vulnerability status can change over time. Circumstances can develop at various stages in the life course which may increase or decrease a woman's risk of disorder. For example, a woman with an abusive childhood may find herself isolated and in a poor marriage at one stage of life, but may develop good friendships and a supportive relationship with a partner at a later stage. By the same token, women *without* backgrounds of childhood neglect or abuse can also find themselves at times vulner-able to depression in adulthood.

Although the route from childhood adversity to adult depression is a disturbingly common pathway, it would be misleading to suggest that this is the only route to adult vulnerability. Poor self-esteem and inadequate support may develop for other reasons at a later stage in life. This is demonstrated in our Adult Risk series of women selected for either low self-esteem or poor support. Here it was found that just under half had experienced *neither* neglect nor abuse in childhood.[15, 16] Stated quite simply, childhood maltreatment makes its impact in adulthood by increasing the chances that a woman will find herself vulnerable or in adverse circumstances in adult life. However, it is conditions in adult life which are crucial to the likelihood of a particular episode of depression occurring at a given time.

CONCLUSION

The quote at the beginning of this chapter emphasises the constraints individuals with a history of abuse develop when forming intimate ties in adulthood. There was certainly evidence of this in our series. However, this only describes part of the picture since the women who experienced neglect or abuse in childhood also experienced more adverse external environments. Vulnerable women were more likely, for example, to be of lower social class, to be poorer, and to be bringing children up in a discordant relationship or else single-handedly. The men they selected to marry were more often unreliable, with a history of psychiatric problems of their own. We found it was the interaction between a fragile inner psychological world (reflected in low self-esteem and poor ability to make relationships), and the challenging circumstances of the outer world (reflected in social and material hardship) that precipitated depression in adulthood.

What is striking in comparing childhood and adult vulnerability is the similarity in contexts. The backdrop for abuse in childhood has several features in common with the adult depressogenic environment. Thus the poverty, marital conflict and psychiatric disorder which accompany childhood neglect and abuse are often reconstructed in adulthood to form not only the conditions for depression in the grown-up child, but also a potential breeding ground for neglect and abuse of the next generation.

We know that depression results from a particular patterning of circumstance, location, personal history, psychological characteristics, and choice of partner or friends. Yet only one part of the jigsaw needs to be out of place for depression to be evaded. Poor support unaccompanied by low self-esteem and vice versa carries substantially lower risk than the two together. Neither factor is potent for depression until activated by life crises. Such vulnerability can be ameliorated at different points in the life course. Breaking just one link in the chain may substantially reduce the likelihood of depression as an outcome.

To return to the life history of the insurance clerk described earlier, there were signs that she was trying to carve out a more positive future for herself by seeking support and learning to trust. She was beginning to nourish her psychological needs and repair the damage inflicted in childhood. For the first time in her life she had disclosed her childhood abuse, initially through a telephone helpline and later in the research interview. The general validation of her experience by such impartial listeners prompted her to seek help in learning to come to terms with her history of abuse and neglect. She felt that the interview itself had helped her to find the courage to start therapy: 'I feel that taking part in this research was like a blessing in disguise. But over the last six weeks I've been able to do a lot of thinking about the whole situation. I realised that if I did not get help pretty soon, things would have only gone from bad to worse. I can only hope that things will get better for me now and that at the end of the day it will all be up to me.'

NOTES

1   Egeland, B. (1993) 'A history of abuse is a major risk factor for abusing the next generation', in Gelles, R.J. and Loseke, D.R. (eds) *Current Controversies on Family Violence*, California, US, London, UK: Sage Publications.
2   Maslow, A. (1973) *The Farther Reaches of Human Nature*, Middlesex: Penguin.

3   *Table 9.1* Premarital pregnancy and neglect in childhood (Loss of
Mother study: those with loss of mother only, N = 139) (% depressed)

Neglect*	Premarital pregnancy		
	Present	Absent	
Present	50 (12/24)	28 (13/47)	
Absent	22 (2/9)	5 (3/59)	
Total	42 (14/33)	15 (16/106)	p < 0.005

* Termed lack of care in the relevant publication.

4   An analysis of the effects of premarital pregnancy is given in: Harris,
T.O., Brown, G.W. and Bifulco, A. (1987) 'Loss of parent in childhood
and adult psychiatric disorder: the role of social class position and
premarital pregnancy', *Psychological Medicine 17*: 163–183.

5   Brown, G.W. and Moran, P.M. (1997) 'Single mothers, poverty and
depression', *Psychological Medicine 27*: 21–33.

6   In the Representative London Women series 27% (78/286) experienced violence in a cohabiting relationship or sexual assault after
age seventeen.

7   Of those with childhood neglect or abuse 44% (36/82) experienced
adult abuse compared with 21% (42/204) without such childhood
experience (p < 0.001).

8   In the Representative London Women series, 31% (24/78) of those
with adult abuse were depressed in the year of interview compared
with 13% (26/208) of those with no adult abuse (p < 0.001).

9   *Table 9.2* Adult abuse, childhood neglect/abuse and depression
(Representative London Women series) (% depressed)

Childhood neglect/abuse	Adult violence/sexual assault		
	Present	Absent	
Present	42 (15/36)	28 (13/46)	NS
Absent	21 (9/42)	8 (13/162)	p < 0.05
Total	31 (24/78)	13 (26/208)	p < 0.001

10   Brown, G.W. and Moran, P. (1994) 'Clinical and psychosocial origins
of chronic depressive episodes, I: a community survey', *British Journal of Psychiatry 165*: 447–456.

11 *Table 9.3* Adult vulnerability and childhood neglect/abuse (Representative London Women series; vulnerability = poor support or low self-esteem)

Neglect/abuse	% adult vulnerability	
Present	71 (58/82)	
Absent	48 (97/204)	
Total	54 (155/286)	p < 0.001

12 Maslow, A. (1973) op. cit. note 2.
13 *Table 9.4* Vulnerability, life crises and onset of case depression (Representative London Women series)* (% depression)

Low self-esteem or poor support	Life crises Present	Absent	Total
Both factors	46 (22/48)	10 (2/21)	35 (24/69)
One factor	16 (7/43)	0 (0/55)	7 (7/98)
None	0 (0/39)	1 (1/97)	1 (1/136)
Total	22 (29/130)	2 (3/173)	11 (32/303) p < 0.001

A different number of women is quoted here from earlier chapters consistent with the prospective part of the study. Appendix I gives details of the samples studied.

14 A detailed analysis of self-esteem, poor support and onset of depression in the representative series is given in: Brown, G.W., Bifulco, A. and Andrews, B. (1990) 'Self-esteem and depression, 3: aetiological issues', *Social Psychiatry and Psychiatric Epidemiology 25*: 235–243.
15 In the Adult Risk series all women were selected for having at least one vulnerability factor of low self-esteem or poor support. Of these although 58% (60/103) had experienced neglect or abuse in childhood this left 42% (43/103) with an absence of childhood abuse and neglect.
16 Bifulco, A., Brown G.W., Moran P., Ball, C. and Campbell, C. (1998) 'Predicting depression in women. The role of past and present vulnerability', *Psychological Medicine* (in press).

Chapter 10

Resilience: escape from risk

... the universal observation that even with the most severe stressors and the most glaring adversities it is unusual for more than half the children to succumb. The same recognition had applied in adults to depression following personal losses and rebuffs. Although the risk of depression following disturbing life events is increased, it is usual for most people not to become depressed.

(Rutter 1985: 598)[1]

Depending on the degree of optimism or pessimism present, the interpretation of a given result in research can be seen in a more or less negative light. For instance, we may be dismayed that as many as a third of children who suffer neglect or abuse develop symptoms of major depression in any one twelve-month period during adult-hood. However, we may be heartened by the fact that the remaining two-thirds of children, despite similar early experience, do *not* become depressed in that year. Even when we consider more severe markers of disorder such as chronic episodes lasting over a year, or depressions which recur over the life course, similar proportions are involved, with around a third succumbing and two-thirds resisting.[2] The reason why some abused children become vulnerable to depression and others escape such risk is bound to be complex and, when full facts are known, would merit volumes of its own. However, the research conducted by our team can at least suggest some factors which appear to promote resilience and survival, and serve as an escape to continued risk for such individuals. Although such analyses represent work in progress with the search for protective factors still very active, we have the means to begin to map out such factors, pointing the way for future models of protectedness and resilience.

The search for positive or protective factors is not as straightforward as might be imagined. In the same way that risk involves a stream of negative circumstance running through life, so resilience or protectedness is likely to follow the same lengthy course. The last chapter demonstrated a chain of related experiences linking childhood neglect and abuse with both early and later adult risk factors. It is the accumulation and escalation of risk over a number of years which make depressive episodes in adulthood a highly probable outcome, not some magical dormant link with childhood across a vacuum devoid of adversity. Thus, at each life stage, risk factors increase the likelihood of further risk factors which ultimately culminate in a disorder. The reverse process can be hypothesised as occurring where protective factors are concerned: at each stage an individual can escape from risk, accumulate protection and reduce the probability of future risks and disorder. Hence the search is not for a single factor which promotes resilience; instead it involves the identification of a variety of factors arising at various life stages, with each factor reducing or protecting against risk combinations, thus breaking the chain of linked disadvantage.

Some such experiences have already been hinted at earlier in this book. We have seen that the presence of supportive others appears to have beneficial effects, for example, where a caring parent has lessened the impact of conflict or poverty in the home. We have also seen how examples of coping in childhood can have ameliorating effects on neglect and abuse. Some children have asserted themselves against their abusers and at times stopped the maltreatment. Other children have taken on extra responsibility and acquired mastery through competent handling of premature adult roles. In our samples we also encountered examples of children finding escape from their difficult conditions through meaningful activity, whether school work, or hobbies such as sport or music. We have seen too, that adult vulnerability to depression is at its most damaging for individuals with *both* poor support and low self-esteem, with depression rates greatly reduced if only one such negative factor is present. Thus by implication, avoiding one such risk can protect against the effects of another.

In this chapter we examine the role that social support, good coping, and meaningful roles and activity play in reducing the risk of depression. In particular we consider the experiences which break the links between childhood neglect/abuse and adult vulnerability to depression. Results are presented in terms of factors which reduce not only the rate of depression in adulthood, but also reduce the vulnerability preceding such disorder, namely low self-esteem or poor support.

The precise effect of a positive factor may vary a great deal. Whereas some factors may simply be associated with less risk, others may have a stronger beneficial effect, only triggered in the presence of neglect and abuse. These are truly protective factors which can actually buffer an individual against the impact of adverse early experiences once they have occurred.[3]

SUPPORT

We have suggested that having one positive source of safety, belonging and identity, could lessen the damage from adversity and increase an individual's psychological 'immune' system, thus inoculating against later adversity. The last chapter discussed the effects of hostile attachments and lack of support in adult life. Here we examine evidence that supportive relationships at various points in the life course can reduce risk.

Childhood support

A supportive figure in childhood may have beneficial effects, not only in conferring a sense of self-worth and 'loveability' to a child, but also in terms of opening up opportunities for later life. These influences may set a child upon a less depressogenic pathway than might otherwise have been expected given the presence of abuse or neglect in early years. Consider, for example, the impact one childhood support figure made on the following woman's life course. As a child she was neglected by both parents, largely because they favoured their only son. This woman was very bright as a child, but because she was a girl she was discouraged from having a career, and was forced to spend much of her time performing domestic chores. She described life with her parents: 'At home we had no books, no paper to draw on, nothing. They never spent any time with me. I remember desperately, desperately wanting to read and since we had no books I'd read anything about the house, even soap packets. My mother knew that I worked hard at school. I got a prize every year. I felt proud that I'd achieved something. My father would never acknowledge it.' She suffered physical abuse from her father throughout childhood and there were constant unfavourable comparisons between her and her brother.

There was however one person in the house who became a support figure. She was an elderly retired woman who lived alone, a lodger in their house. She became attached to the child, and confronted the father when he beat the girl. The retired woman spent much time with her, took her out for day trips, bought her books to read, and took an interest in her school work. 'She was an inspiration to me. She was my voice as a child. She encouraged me to go to college and get a good education.' At eighteen the woman successfully applied to college to train for teaching which she then took up as her career. We can only guess at what might have happened had this child not received affection, concern and encouragement from the supportive, retired lady. She may have succumbed to the teenage risks of pregnancy, early marriage or entrapment in the abusive parental home, all outcomes which we know to be likely to result in adult depressive disorder.

A second example of how a childhood support figure can have a beneficial effect is one that has been quoted earlier in the chapter concerning physical abuse. It illustrates how one woman overcame her childhood abuse, not through educational opportunities, but through the advice given by an older woman. The woman's encouraging words helped the girl to cope with her physically abusive father. 'She kept saying to me "If you let your dad carry on like this, he's going to rule your life" and I didn't want that. I confronted him and he never struck me after that. I realised she had been right, I had to stand my ground.'

The presence of a positive relationship in childhood as a possible protection against the damage inflicted by neglectful or abusive parent figures was examined in our sample of Sisters. We defined support in childhood as the presence of a person to whom the child could go for help, and to whom the child could confide their problems, or else someone who acted as a role model for the child, whom the child looked up to. This encompassed relatives (excluding parents), teachers, family friends and even peers. We found that whereas only 19 per cent with such support in childhood became depressed as adults, this compared with 39 per cent with no childhood support.[4] This does imply a positive effect, but the real test of its protective nature was to assess whether such support reduced depression when neglect and abuse were present. There was indeed evidence of this, with 28 per cent of those with neglect/abuse and childhood support being depressed in the interview year compared with 42 per cent of women with similar abuse but no support. In the absence of neglect or abuse the figures were 12 per cent for those with childhood support becoming depressed and 31 per cent of those with no such support, respectively.

Teenage support

Another critical life stage when circumstances can lead to an escalation of risk is during teenage years when experiences for young women such as unplanned pregnancy can have an entrapping effect. We therefore considered whether support with such a teenage crisis could reduce the risk of future vulnerability. There was some evidence of this in the descriptions we obtained at interview. One illustration was from a young woman with an adverse childhood who became pregnant at sixteen while still at school. She had tried asking her mother for contraceptive advice but none was forthcoming in a context of parental neglect and physical abuse. Her boyfriend was highly supportive over the pregnancy, and since neither of them wanted her to have a termination he supported her decision in keeping the baby. He asked her to marry him and they planned where they would live while he found a job. To the girl's surprise her parents were also supportive. She and her boyfriend moved into a hostel for teenage mothers for the first six months of the baby's life, after which they were offered a council flat. She was delighted with her new baby, the marriage and their new accommodation. The marriage continued happily for seven years and she did not suffer depression during this time. Without the support of her partner at the time of the pregnancy, depression would have been a much more probable immediate and future outcome, as our results testify.

Although we had only descriptive evidence of such support having an impact for teenage pregnancy, when we examined *any* prior stressful pregnancy, whether teenage or not, we found that partner's support with the pregnancy did have a modest effect in lessening the rate of later adult vulnerability at interview. We defined a stressful pregnancy as one where there were ongoing difficulties with health, housing or relationships, or where the pregnancy was unplanned or resulted in miscarriage or stillbirth. Most pregnancies in teenage years qualified as stressful in this sense. Of those with a stressful pregnancy and partner support, 60 per cent went on to develop later adult vulnerability (in terms of low self-esteem or poor support in the year of interview) compared with as many as 80 per cent of those without such support.[5]

Adult support

From the discussion in the last chapter it can be seen that inadequate support can render a person vulnerable to the impact of a life crisis, with depression as a consequence. We therefore considered the positive role of support in adult life and assessed its ability to act as a buffer against the effects of such unpleasant events. Thus, if vulnerability to depression was conferred by inadequate support in the form of absent or hostile relationships, we questioned whether the presence of a supportive close relationship protected against the onset of depression in the face of a crisis. Several examples attesting to the protective effects of a supportive close relationship were evident in out surveys. An illustration of this is provided by the woman described earlier who went on to train as a teacher with the encouragement of the retired lady lodger. She was experiencing a difficult time in her marriage when we interviewed her. A few months before the interview she had became unexpectedly pregnant. Her husband had proved particularly unsupportive and unrespon-sive. She was very upset because she realised a termination was inevitable due to their financial circumstances and the burden of caring for the large family they already had. Yet her commitment to parenthood was very high. 'The pregnancy was totally unexpected. I just cannot understand it. I was so shocked. It was a terrible experience. Women who have terminations are in a real dilemma.'

Although her husband was unsupportive, she had a particularly close friendship with a woman she has known some years and who had moved to Scotland. When faced with the decision to terminate the pregnancy, she confided in her friend who immediately came down to London to help her over the crisis. 'I trust and respect her. I do have other friends but they rely more on me than I do on them. This particular friend is my "agony aunt" I suppose as well as a great friend. She really helped me cope and supported my decision.' Despite an unsupportive response from her partner, this woman did not become depressed after this crisis.

In our analysis we found that support from a close tie in a crisis such as this reduced risk of depression: 12 per cent of those with such support compared with 40 per cent without became depressed.

This held even for women whose partners failed to provide ongoing support prior to the crisis. Among such women 26 per cent became depressed after receiving other help during the crisis compared with 45 per cent who had neither ongoing partner support nor crisis support.[6] The effect also held for those who reported continuous support from partner: only 6 per cent became depressed compared to 30 per cent of those whose partners had been supportive but let them down unexpectedly at the time of the crisis.

We also examined the effects of support among the Adult Risk series of women who were selected for being vulnerable adults. This group proved to have a very high risk of depression. Of the total sample, over one in three became depressed during a twelve-month period, and among those who encountered a life crisis, as many as half became depressed.[7] However, one factor which proved protective was prior ability to make and maintain relationships successfully. This assessment was arrived at by examining a range of potential support figures available, not only partner. Thus, although a woman might experience problems in a particular ongoing relationship with partner, friend or child, she could still be considered 'good' at making relationships if she had other close friends and confidants. Such women were only half as likely to become depressed (24 per cent versus 46 per cent), despite being handicapped by ongoing vulnerability and crises.[8]

GOOD COPING

Good coping was another factor examined as a possible protection against adversity at different points in the life course. It was defined mainly in terms of competence in handling life crises, as indicated by taking initiative, planning ahead, practical problem-tackling, and taking responsibility for the problem. We hypothesised that, when faced with difficult circumstances, such masterful coping would ameliorate the problem and ultimately reduce its unpleasant consequences. In addition it would allow positive reappraisal of the problem, allowing greater optimism and reducing the chance of depression developing.

Childhood coping

Although children have a great deal less power than adults they can nevertheless be highly proactive, displaying capability and competence when circumstances require it. A recent book about childhood heroism in the Second World War indicates the level of courage some children can muster when faced with arduous conditions: 'A Time to Fight Back focuses on the experiences of six children caught in the web of World War II. In France, a deaf mute rescued an American fighter pilot whose plane had been shot down. In Belgium a child distributed a clandestine newspaper and in Scotland a young teenager wrote of her fears of a German invasion of her island. Of the other three children the first spent years in hiding, the second was a prisoner at Auschwitz, and the third was a four-year-old victim of bombing raids over Germany. Each story is unique. Each is a tale of remarkable courage.'[9] This quote cites examples of masterful childhood coping in the face of extreme circumstances, but also illustrates how coping is a difficult strategy to assess, since it is usually only fully activated by adverse conditions. In the absence of adversity it is unclear how a child might cope when fully challenged. Thus coping cannot be gauged equally for all individuals at any one time, but is dependent on their situation.

There were many instances of good coping or mastery among the women who suffered neglect or abuse in childhood. Examples have been quoted in earlier chapters, particularly in relation to role-reversal which required taking responsibility for family members, and also in relation to physical abuse, where some children made a spirited stand against their abuser resulting in a reduction, and sometimes a total cessation, of the abuse. One example of such coping was provided by a women who retaliated against the physical abuse she suffered at the hands of her stepfather when she was only ten years old: 'For quite a while he succeeded in making me feel worthless, and then something inside me just snapped, and I just had this feeling that I had to survive him, that I had to wait until I was old enough to walk away. I had to stop him from doing it. That's why I was the only one out of the four sisters that ever stood up to him, that ever fought with him physically. I'd resigned myself to the fact that there was only one person that was going to get me out of this and that was me – my only weapon was myself. That's what I was built for and aimed for.'

Such good coping was often associated with a sense of responsibility and protectiveness for others as discussed in the earlier chapter on role-reversal. The child in the above example also had the courage to disclose her physical abuse to a teacher, and often took beatings instead of her sisters, to protect them. In addition she coped with her own material care when her mother failed to do so: 'I discovered as a small child that as soon as you were old enough to stand on a chair and butter a piece of bread that you wouldn't go hungry.'

One effect of good coping is to prevent a problem from developing. Hence rather than stopping ongoing abuse, some children managed to prevent its occurrence in the first place. This can be seen in the following example, where a girl avoided a sexual assault through masterful handling of a potentially damaging situation: 'I had an experience when I was in hospital aged ten. There was this man who was going round abusing the other children and he came into my room and he told me he was a vicar. He was talking to me and he kept asking me if he could tickle me. I said ''No, you mustn't do that'', because my dad had already explained that my body was my own and that I mustn't let anyone touch it if I didn't want them to. I got a bit frightened. I rang the bell for the nurse and he left. He didn't touch me. Then when my dad and mum came that night to see me, I explained to them what happened and my dad told the police. Apparently when the police came, they said that all the children on the ward had been abused, I was the only one that this man hadn't abused. He was a hospital porter and he was sent to prison for 18 months. I was the only witness because I was ten, and all the others were small children, too young to give evidence. He had abused nine of them. I was the only one that said ''no''.'

This same child was also responsible for reducing the negative consequences of other adversity in her life. When her parents fought violently, for example, she regularly called the police to contain their fighting. She also managed to arrange for herself to be re-admitted into a children's home when the situation in her parental home deteriorated. We can only speculate on the origins of such mastery. This woman was close to her caring father but suffered neglect and physical abuse at the hands of her erratic and mentally disordered mother.

We found good coping modestly related to a lower rate of subsequent adult depression only for those with lower levels of family problems, where neglect or abuse were absent or only present to 'mild' levels. Among the latter group none with good coping became depressed in adulthood compared with 17 per cent of those with poorer coping. But good coping in childhood was not sufficient to counteract the effects of abuse. Among women who had been neglected or abused as children similar rates of adult depression were found for both good and poor childhood copers.[10] Thus, childhood coping was not powerful enough to protect women from developing depression later in life. What we could not gauge was how many abuses had been averted or made less severe because of early masterful action, thus masking its true role. Neither could we assess how often such mastery had protected others from damage, either younger siblings or at times helpless parents.

Teenage coping

In the last chapter the long-term risks of unsupported teenage pregnancy were discussed. One important finding from the Loss of Mother series was that an individual's method of coping with such a pregnancy influenced her risk of future depression. Ineffective coping was defined in terms of passivity and acquiescence resulting in entrapping arrangements, such as being forced to marry the father of the baby despite having no previous intention to do so, or an unplanned phase of single parenthood, having failed to consider the option of termination. Effective coping involved avoiding these traps by use of planned strategies such as having a termination or only marrying the father if this had previously been planned. Of those with ineffective coping 59 per cent became depressed in the study period compared with 25 per cent of those with effective coping, and 15 per cent of those with no such difficult pregnancy.[11,12]

Other examples of masterful coping in teenage years emerged from descriptions of leaving home. Consider the woman described earlier who consciously planned to defy her physically abusive stepfather: 'I knew I had to put up with it legally until my sixteenth birthday, and on the morning of my sixteenth birthday I jumped up, with a suitcase I had already packed and said "Right, you can't keep me any longer, and you can't force me to stay away from my real dad now, I'm legally old enough, I'm going" and I did just that.' She travelled over a hundred miles to London and through her own determination tracked down her father whom she had not seen since she was eight years old.

In the Sisters series, 46 per cent who coped masterfully with leaving home encountered vulnerability later as adults compared with 65 per cent of those who left home in an unplanned manner. This effect was almost entirely restricted to those with prior neglect or abuse. Among this group only 42 per cent developed later vulnerability compared with 73 per cent who showed poorer coping skills when leaving an abusive home. For those without such early adversity, masterful coping did not affect future vulnerability.[13] Thus when leaving home, good coping skills acted as a protective factor, buffering against the effects of neglect and abuse to reduce future vulnerability.

Adult coping

Coping well with life crises in adulthood also reduced risk of depression. An illustration of this is the teacher described earlier who was supported by her friend in Scotland when she found herself pregnant. She arranged some counselling for herself and her husband, and organised a termination early on in the pregnancy. She also tried to make the best of the situation by reappraising it in a more positive light, and managed to retain some optimism: 'I did tell myself it could have been worse. I thought, well if I lived in a different country I wouldn't have any choice. I would have to have the baby whether I liked it or not. Yes, it could be worse, I have got the choice. I've even got my own financial resources so I could have done it privately if I'd wanted. There are people who aren't as fortunate as I am, who can't take steps quickly to sort themselves out.' This 'downplaying' of the negative consequences related to a lower risk of depression following a severely unpleasant event. In our Representative London Women series we found that none of the women with this cognitive strategy became depressed after a life crisis compared with 24 per cent of other women.[14] Among vulnerable women the effect still held: none of the 'downplayers' became depressed compared with 33 per cent of the remainder. This style of cognitive reappraisal was associated with higher practical problem-tackling, lower helplessness, higher optimism, higher self-esteem and greater utilisation of support.[15]

Among the women selected for vulnerability in our Adult Risk series, we examined good coping in terms of a range of responses to crises involving either downplaying the negative aspects of a crisis, retaining hope of its resolution, or else having high practical mastery. We then compared the outcomes of these women who coped well with those who used other strategies when faced with a life crisis in the year we saw them. We found the presence of the positive coping more than halved the rate of depression when compared to the use of other coping.[16] This effect held even for those with childhood neglect or abuse where 30 per cent with good coping became depressed compared with 59 per cent with moderate or poor coping.

MEANINGFUL ROLES

Another type of factor we considered as a possible protection against vulnerability and depression was the presence of meaningful or rewarding roles. It seemed that such roles could have a positive effect in several ways. First they could be beneficial in providing a sense of identity and a source of self-esteem. Second, they might act as a source of pleasure and hope, and distract a woman from the adversity that might be present in other domains of her life.

Childhood and teenage meaningful roles

In their accounts of childhood, many of the abused women commented that they had preferred being at school to being at home. Indeed, they preferred being *anywhere* to being at home. It seemed that school or other extra-curricular activities offered a welcome escape from the abusive household. Involvement in such activities also took their minds off painful home experiences and gave them opportunities for developing a sense of achievement. Some became very proficient at school activities, whether academic or non-academic. We have already seen in an earlier example how the woman who received support from the elderly lodger managed to take up further education and use her academic abilities as a route out of vulnerability. There were several other examples of this nature. Another woman's sporting achievements helped her to escape from an abusive home environment on a deprived northern housing estate. Due to her skill at rowing she was able to move to London and achieve a place in the national team, thus permanently changing her life for the better. Rowing not only represented an escape route from an abusive environment, it also opened up social and material opportunities she would otherwise never have had access to. Despite childhood neglect and abuse, she developed a strong sense of purpose and good self-esteem which protected her against depression in later years.

When we examined academic achievement at school in the Sisters series, we found it resulted generally in a much reduced rate of later adult vulnerability defined by low self-esteem or poor support. Thus whereas half of those who gained GCEs at 'O' or 'A' level were vulnerable at the time of interview, this compared with as many as 71 per cent of those without. Such competence at school was much less common among women with childhood neglect or abuse: only 43 per cent of those with abusive childhoods achieved well at school compared with 63 per cent of other children. However, an examination of the effects of such competence among those with childhood adversity showed no protective effect against abuse: its beneficial effect worked solely for those with no childhood abuse or neglect.[17] However, this does inform us of additional deprivation associated with abuse in childhood. We have seen in earlier chapters how the effects of neglect and role-reversal in particular impede the child's success at school through parental non-involvement and the burden of domestic work placed on the child. It appears that such disinterest hampers children in educational and career terms, as well as emotional and social terms.

In addition to school achievement, women described how part-time work prior to school-leaving gave them confidence and a sense of purpose. One woman gave an account of the independence and sense of identity she derived from her early commitment to work: 'I started working as a child when I was about eleven and full-time when I was sixteen. I worked for a newsagent, filling up shelves and helping over the counter a couple of nights a week and on Saturdays. I've been a milk girl in my day, up at the crack of dawn delivering milk, and I also worked in a cafe. Some of the money I managed to keep, especially in the cafe because of the tips that my father didn't know about. But most of my money he would ask if he could borrow it, but I never saw it again after that. But it gave me some independence, some sense that I could do something for myself and maybe one day get out.'

Clearly, having a job provided her with material and emotional resources which helped her to cope with life under her parent's roof. However, she was unable to escape from her abusive home until some years later. She had planned to move away by taking up further education but was thwarted by her infrequent school attendance and subsequent poor exam results. She worked as a secretary at sixteen while still living in the parental home. She then moved out of her parents' home at eighteen and lived with a friend, but had to return home to support her younger sister who had made a suicide attempt. Again she felt trapped, but eventually managed to change jobs to become a lawyer's assistant, which offered opportunities of promotion and further training. With the help of her new employer she managed to buy her own flat and leave home at twenty-three. She finally achieved the independence she craved and kept depression at bay.

Adult meaningful roles

Just as children and teenagers derive beneficial effects from rewarding roles and activities, so too do adults for much the same reason. Paid employment or other meaningful roles can detract from the challenges faced in a depressogenic environment involving marital conflict, problems with children or loneliness. Such roles may also boost confidence and self-esteem, thus reducing vulnerability to depression. This was certainly true in the case of the woman described above, who derived a great sense of achievement from success at work and also from owning her own flat. 'The turning point for me was getting my own flat because then I didn't have to answer to anybody. I felt like that's when my life really began. I didn't get any assistance from anybody. My dad said I wouldn't make it on my own: "I'll give it a month and you'll be back." I didn't ask for any help, I didn't want any help, I didn't want any hand-outs. It's important to know what you're doing, and I feel that I do. I'm particularly good at my job and can run the house, handle the money and organise my life.' Through fulfilment in her work and personal life she had managed to keep her self-esteem relatively intact despite her abusive childhood, and thus acquired some protection from depression.

Employment was shown to protect against depression even among women with vulnerability. Research by George Brown and Tirril Harris in Camberwell in the 1970s showed that women with part- or full-time employment had half the rate of depression of those not working.[18, 19] Further analysis showed it was indeed protective against the ill-effects of poor support: only 13 per cent of those who were in employment and had poor support were depressed compared with 30 per cent of those who were unemployed with similarly poor support. Therefore employment can be seen as an alternative investment to close relationships for some women insofar as it protects against depression. There was also some evidence to support the notion that employment countered vulnerability to depression by boosting self-esteem. For married mothers in the Representative series 13 per cent in full-time work had low self-esteem compared to 25 per cent in part-time work and 29 per cent with no work.[20]

The protective effects of paid employment are easier to understand for childless women and for those with few alternative roles. Where mothers are concerned the picture becomes more complicated, since the burden from competing roles needs to be taken into account. When employment outside the home was examined among working-class *mothers* in the Representative series we found that part-time work alone was protective against depression with full-time working mothers having a higher rate of depression by comparison.[21] When their working life was examined in more detail, mothers in full-time work were found to suffer more work strain than those in part-time employment. This was defined in terms of the level of conflict felt between their motherhood and work roles, as well as the level of unrewarding work conditions they encountered. This was particularly true for single mothers.[22] Therefore employment for women cannot be seen as unequivocally beneficial where the prevention of depression is concerned: much depends on the context of competing responsibilities as well as the nature of the work experience itself. The fewer other roles, the greater the positive features of the employment as a source of self-esteem, the more it is likely to buffer against depression.

Success in other areas of life besides employment or support can increase feelings of self-worth. For example, the woman described earlier who had trained as a teacher told us that although she had derived much satisfaction from her job, she gave up paid employment in order to look after her four young children. She had very high commitment to her mothering role which gave her a strong sense of identity: 'I love my kids, I adore them, they're wonderful. I love being a mum. I had nothing when I was a child and I don't want my children to experience that. I do find it hard looking after all four but I feel in the end its all worthwhile. I love doing things with the children and having fun with them. They give me a lot of pleasure and a lot of grief. I am here trying to be the best mother I can. I feel I have a purpose in life.'

Achieving qualifications later in life also bolstered self-esteem and thus reduced vulnerability to depression. Teenage pregnancy often curtailed educational opportunities at the appropriate life stage, but sometimes women returned to education and made up for lost time. The woman described earlier who got pregnant at sixteen had in recent years managed to undertake her very first qualification. She had completed a course in childcare, and was extremely proud of her exam results: 'It was the first time I had ever achieved anything like that on my own. I was so proud of the certificate, I put it up on the kitchen fridge and just looking at it made me feel good.' This contributed to her feelings of self-esteem, which had been chronically low since childhood, and thus represented a step in the direction of reducing her future risk for depression.

In the Representative series of mothers, women who reported a high degree of 'meaningfulness of life' were found to have greater feelings of control, satisfaction and positive self-esteem compared to others. These factors in turn were associated with enjoyable communication with partner, children and work colleagues, and a high degree of social contacts. Positive factors such as these mirror the negative ones which confer vulnerability to depression. For married/cohabiting women, rewarding relationships with partner and children contributed to a positive self-image and buffered against low self-esteem.[23] For single mothers high self-esteem and meaningfulness of life were also correlated with financial security.[24] Thus meaningful involvement of one kind or another has multiple benefits, many of which contribute to the avoidance of risk for depression. Such involvements and activities can interrupt the stream of negative experiences which leads to disorder.

CONCLUSION

Just as the analysis outlined in this book has sought to draw together a variety of risks in a relatively simple framework, the same exercise needs to be undertaken with regard to positive life experiences. The positive factors described above tend to cluster: those with better support tended to be better copers, and these in turn tended to have more meaningful roles. It may prove difficult to disentangle the pathways linking these factors. As with adverse experiences which tend to come in droves rather than singly, so positive factors gather momentum and can act cumulatively. The woman who started work as a lawyer's assistant gained support, sense of identity, self-esteem and financial independence from her job. The woman who was helped with her teenage pregnancy by a supportive boyfriend simultaneously acquired a home, husband and baby, and escaped from an abusive household. The woman whose supportive lodger encouraged her to go to college planned her escape from her abusive home and acquired an education and career. Each of these women tells a tale of survival, although none emerged completely unscathed. At times each of them was plagued with self-doubt, worry about their capacities as parents, partners or friends, and harboured resentments about the past. Encouragingly, many expressed a determination to break the cycle of disadvantage for future generations.

NOTES

1 Rutter, M. (1985) 'Resilience in the face of adversity. Protective factors and resistance to psychiatric disorder', *British Journal of Psychiatry 147*: 598–611.

2 *Table 10.1* Chronicity of depression and repeated episodes in adult life by childhood neglect/abuse (Sisters series)

Neglect/abuse	% chronic depression	% recurrent depression
Present	39 (42/108)	33 (36/108)
Absent	19 (17/90)	14 (13/90)
	$p < 0.005$	$p < 0.005$

3 Luthar, S. (1993) 'Annotation: methodological and conceptual issues in research on child resilience', *Journal of Child Psychology and Psychiatry 34*: 441–453.

4 *Table 10.2* Neglect/abuse, childhood support and depression (Sisters series) (% depressed)

Neglect/abuse	Support in childhood		
	Present	Absent	
Present	28 (18/65)	42 (18/43)	
Absent	12 (9/77)	31 (4/13)	
Total	19 (27/142)	39 (22/56)	$p < 0.01$

5 *Table 10.3* Partner support with stressful pregnancy and later adult vulnerability (Sisters series; those with a stressful pregnancy, N = 83) (% later vulnerability)

Partner support	Any stressful pregnancy
Present	60 (26/43)
Absent	80 (32/40)
	$p < 0.10$

6   *Table 10.4* Conflictful unsupportive partner relationship, subsequent crisis support and depression (Representative London Women, tested prospectively; Married/cohabiting only, N = 97) (% depressed)

Conflictful relationship prior to crisis	Crisis support after event	
	Present	*Absent*
Absent	6 (3/48)	30 (3/10)
Present	26 (5/19)	45 (9/20)
Total	12 (8/67)	40 (12/30) p < 0.005

7   Among the Adult Risk series (selected for either low self-esteem or conflict in close relationships and lack of support) 37% (39/105) became depressed over a 14-month period. For those with a severe event 48% (35/73) became depressed compared with 13% (4/32) of those without (p < 0.005).

8   *Table 10.5* Ability to make relationships and depression among vulnerable women (Adult Risk series; tested prospectively, 2 missing values)

Ability to make relationships	% depressed
Good	24 (10/42)
Poor	46 (28/61)
Total	37 (38/103) p < 0.025

9   From the jacket of Pettit, J. (1995) *A Time to Fight Back. True Stories of Children's Resistance During World War 2*, Basingstoke: Macmillan's Children's Books.

10   *Table 10.6* Coping in childhood, neglect/abuse and depression (Sisters series)

Neglect/abuse	Childhood coping	
	Good	*Moderate/poor*
	% depressed	
Present	33 (9/27)	34 (27/80)
Absent	0 (0/13)	17 (13/78)
Total	23 (9/40)	25 (40/158) NS

11 *Table 10.7* Premarital pregnancy and coping (Loss of Mother series)

Coping with pregnancy	% depressed
Poor coping	59 (10/17)
Good coping	25 (4/16)
No premarital pregnancy	15 (16/106)
	p < 0.001, 2 df

12 Harris, T.O., Brown, G.W. and Bifulco, A. (1987) 'Loss of parent in childhood and adult psychiatric disorder: the role of social class position and premarital pregnancy', *Psychological Medicine 17*: 163–183.

13 *Table 10.8* Coping with leaving home and adult vulnerability (Sisters series; N = 184, 14 women living at home at interview) (% adult vulnerability)

Neglect/abuse	Coping with leaving home		
	Good	Moderate/poor	
Present	42 (10/24)	73 (55/75)	p < 0.025
Absent	54 (7/13)	56 (40/72)	NS
Total	46 (17/37)	65 (95/147)	p < 0.10

14 *Table 10.9* Cognitive coping and depression (Representative London Women series; those with a severe event at first follow-up interview, N = 147, 3 missing values) (% depressed)

Adult vulnerability	Downplaying the crisis	
	Yes	No
Present	0 (0/13)	33 (26/80)
Absent	0 (0/5)	10 (5/49)
Total	0 (0/18)	24 (31/129) p < 0.10

15 Bifulco, A. and Brown, G.W. (1996) 'Cognitive coping response to crises and onset of depression', *Journal of Social Psychiatry and Psychiatric Epidemiology 31*: 163–172.

16 *Table 10.10* Coping with recent crises, childhood neglect/abuse and depression (Adult Risk series; vulnerable women only with severe event at follow-up) (% depressed)

Neglect/abuse	Coping with recent crises	
	Good*	Moderate/poor
Present	30 (3/10)	59 (24/41)
Absent	9 (1/11)	45 (13/29)
Total	19 (4/21)	53 (37/70) $p < 0.025$

* Good coping = either high downplaying, high mastery or high optimism

17 *Table 10.11* Academic achievement at school and adult vulnerability (Sisters series; 2 missing values) (% adult vulnerability)

Neglect/abuse	Academic achievement		
	High	Low	
Present	63 (29/46)	68 (41/60)	
Absent	40 (23/57)	76 (25/33)	
Total	50 (52/103)	71 (66/93)	$p < 0.01$

18 *Table 10.12* Employment in year of interview, support and depression (Camberwell series; see Brown and Harris 1978: 181) (% depressed)

Support	Employed	Unemployed	
Good	3 (5/170)	5 (6/121)	NS
Poor	13 (11/88)	30 (15/50)	$p < 0.025$
Total	6 (16/258)	12 (21/171)	$p < 0.05$

19 Brown, G.W. and Harris, T.O. (1978) *Social Origins of Depression*, London: Tavistock.

20 *Table 10.13* Employment and self-esteem (Representative London Women series; married only)

Employment	% low self-esteem
Full-time	13 (7/52)
Part-time	25 (27/108)
No work	29 (32/112)
	$p < 0.10$

21 *Table 10.14* Employment and depression among mothers (Representative London Women series; women with a severe event at follow-up, N = 150)

Employment	% depression
Full-time	34 (13/88)
Part-time	8 (4/50)
Not working	21 (13/62)
	$p < 0.01$, 2 df

22 Brown, G.W. and Bifulco, A. (1990) 'Motherhood, employment and the development of depression. A replication of a finding?' *British Journal of Psychiatry 156*: 169–179.

23 Brown, G.W., Bifulco, A., Veiel, H. and Andrews, B. (1990) 'Self-esteem and depression, 2: social correlates of self-esteem', *Social Psychiatry and Psychiatric Epidemiology 25*: 225–234.

24 Brown, G.W. and Moran, P.M. (1997) 'Single mothers, poverty and depression', *Psychological Medicine 27*: 21–33.

Chapter 11

Conclusion: the century of the child

This vision of the 'century of the child' attracted reformers for
most of the first half of the century. Their overriding aim was to
map out a territory called 'childhood' and put in place frontier
posts which would prevent too early escape from what was seen
as desirably a garden of delight. Within this garden children
would be cared for and acquire the 'habit of happiness'.

(Cunningham 1995: 164)[1]

AN HISTORICAL PERSPECTIVE

We have witnessed a dramatic evolution in the treatment of children
over the last hundred years, with children having been increasingly
seen as vulnerable and in need of protection, surveillance and
control by adults. Great social and political significance has been
placed on saving children from the 'nasty infections of adulthood
such as sex, violence and commerce'.[2] Energetic philanthropy at the
end of the last century led to dramatic improvements in childcare
and protection. Factory and Education Acts protected children from
punishing work conditions and enclosed them in the world of
school, while criminal legislation halted the use of barbarous penal-
ties for children including transportation, imprisonment and death.
Such developments have led to the optimistic view of the twentieth
century as the 'century of the child'.

Child abuse as discussed here is not a particularly modern con-
cept, having emerged in the thirty years or so prior to the First
World War.[3] Its emergence has been paralleled by the introduction
of organisations representing the needs of children. These include
bodies such as the NSPCC which, by 1910, had 250 inspectors who
investigated over 50,000 complaints about the treatment of children.

In the period after the First World War the international 'Save the Children Fund' formed by Eglantyne Jebb, drew up a simple declaration of children's rights which was adopted by the League of Nations in 1924.

Concerns for the rights of the child have increasingly come to the fore in the second half of the twentieth century. Our image of children as vulnerable individuals in need of parental protection has gradually been altered to incorporate the notion of children as autonomous beings whose voices must be heard. The 1989 United Nations Convention on the Rights of the Child, for example, not only provided for child protection but also for the right of the child to contribute in any decision that may affect his or her life. Now children in the UK and US have the right to bring legal proceedings against their own parents, an indication of the shifting power balance between parent and child.

PREVENTION OF ABUSE IN CHILDHOOD

The primary aim of this book has been to demonstrate links between maltreatment in childhood and risk of adult depression. Thus the prevention of child abuse obviously represents one strategy for reducing adult depression. In 1996 the NSPCC established the National Commission into the Prevention of Child Abuse, whose report, based on the contribution of some 10,000 people, has already been referred to extensively in this book. It optimistically concludes that 'nearly all forms of child abuse can be prevented'.[4] The report contains a wide-ranging list of recommendations involving areas of legislation, employment, finance, education, health and social service provision, as well as media and research coverage. To give some indication of the types of strategies for preventing abuse recommended in the report, the following are included: the appointment of a Minister for Children; the facilitation of methods for children to give evidence in court against abusers; tighter regulation of employment of those who work with children in nursery schools and children's homes; training of teachers to spot the indicators of abuse and to reduce bullying; training of all police officers in the area of child protection so that suspected child abuse situations can be identified early; encouragement of individuals such as neighbours to come forward if abuse of a child is suspected; and education in parenting both in school and post-school. It also recommends further research into both the context in which abuse occurs and into characteristics of abusers. In terms of helping children to cope with abuse when it does occur, we would underline the following from our own findings: teaching adults to recognise abuse with procedures for intervening and making it easier for children to access support from adults, greater help for children in disclosing abuse and increased opportunities in school for acquiring self-esteem, coping and life-skills to help overcome the effects of abuse.

Although the enforcement of many of the changes required to combat and prevent abuse is costly, this is not necessarily any more than the estimated £1 billion already spent annually on providing support and services for children who have been abused. Supporters of preventative strategies argue that the cost could be drastically reduced if resources were channelled into the prevention of abuse. It has been estimated, for example, that if currently the problems of a mere 10 per cent of adults in mental health care and prison result from childhood abuse, then £348 million annually would be saved on services if the abuse had been prevented. The savings would be even greater if one counts the cost of services for abused children such as special education, residential and psychiatric care.

However, as the Commission's report points out, a significant reduction in child abuse cannot take place without a radical shift in society's attitudes towards children. While the Commission reports that abuse is largely preventable, it emphasises that this is only 'provided the will to do so is there'. Thus a move towards a more child-orientated society is required before effective protection of children can take place. The report stresses the importance of children's rights and their need to be heard. A shift towards this position has been witnessed in recent years with the introduction of legislation protecting the rights of children. As children's writer Michael Rosen points out, the connection between the rights of children and their abuse has long been unrecognised: 'There is something intractably circular about a culture that denies children power and produces people who abuse children. This abuse is rightly condemned, yet is usually seen as unrelated to the ways the culture controls and limits children.'[5]

PREVENTION OF ADULT RISK FACTORS

As well as examining possible means of preventing child abuse, we also need to simultaneously consider the possibilities of preventing later risks for depression further along the risk pathway. For many, damage has already been inflicted by the time they reach early adulthood when the experience of adult vulnerability and the impact of life stressors need to be combated. Strategies for the prevention of future psychopathology are possible at three different levels and stages in the pathway to depression. The first involves reducing the prevalence of psychosocial risk factors. Thus in terms of the model described here this would involve reducing rates of experiences such as teenage unplanned pregnancy, violence in cohabiting relationships, or the frequency or intensity with which life crises occur. The second strategy for prevention concerns preparing individuals to face psychosocial stress when it does occur. Thus improving an individual's self-esteem, coping resources or quality of relationships prior to encountering a particular stressor would make for better preparation and 'inoculation' against the impact of the stressor. The third strategy for prevention involves taking action at the time of the stressor to try to ameliorate its effects and buffer against some of its worst impact. Thus providing additional support and counselling for people experiencing crises would aid coping and influence appraisal of crises in a positive way. This may serve to reduce the impact of life crises and thereby lower risk of disorder.

Since we cannot 'undo' the childhood neglect and abuse which have already occurred in the lives of people who are adults today, these later types of prevention need to be undertaken in conjunction with prevention of current neglect or abuse to children. All are possible, and indeed are already being tackled through the ongoing work of a variety of charitable, voluntary sector and government agencies, utilising a range of educative, psychotherapeutic, 'befriending' or self-help schemes. In terms of the model of depression presented here we see any intervention benefiting from a specific 'theory-driven' focus based on factors we have covered including self-esteem, coping skills and planning, ability to relate to others and utilisation of support. Ideally, such preventative strategies would be available at several points in the life-course in order to reduce future risk of disorder for those with adverse childhood experience.

These preventative strategies should ideally be available from earliest years. Not only would they help children combat and cope with abusive experiences but they might have particular beneficial impact for teenagers in influencing their choices and opportunities for the future. In our series of Sisters, 30 per cent of those with neglect or abuse reported already having suffered a clinical depression by the end of their teenage years, treble the rate among those without such childhood adversity. Thus tackling the problem effectively at an early life stage is desirable. The earlier the preventative action, the sooner an individual can be set on a positive pathway into adulthood, to form supportive relationships, feel good about themselves, and ultimately be in a better position to care for their own children.

OUR ETHICAL POSITION AS RESEARCHERS

Despite the effort and concern which go into research such as ours, at times the role of researcher is criticised – we neither treat distressed individuals, nor do we attempt to remedy the problems which have given rise to their distress. In this sense research is often viewed as a less worthwhile occupation than the more 'practical' professions such as psychiatry or social work. As our team is based in a university rather than a treatment centre and our researchers are not qualified practitioners, we are unable to offer direct help. We are careful to make this clear to participants at the commencement of our interviews. However, there have been occasions when women we have interviewed have asked us for assistance. In these cases we have been able to refer women back to their own general practitioner, or provide them with information about local facilities such as treatment centres or self-help groups. On some occasions we have been able to provide more direct help. Once our research interview has been completed, we have on occasion written to local authorities, for example, in support of women's applications to be rehoused away from violent partners or substandard housing conditions. In this way our research has been able to substantiate women's claim that the circumstances they find themselves in are detrimental to their own mental health as well as that of their children.

ABUSE AND PARENTING

One of the effects of increased vigilance over the protection of children has been the scrutiny of the role of parenthood. From the 1920s and 1930s a scientific approach to bringing up children has been advocated through a number of books and magazines aimed at parents. First the virtues of behaviourism were extolled with the emphasis on establishing what Truby King in 1937 called the 'regularity of habits' with use of rewards and punishments to condition the infants' behaviour. This was followed after the Second World War by a more relaxed recommendation by Dr Spock that parents should enjoy parenting, be more permissive with their children and more attentive to their needs.

These changing conceptions of childcare across the century have led to apparently contradictory parenting requirements. Once the function of parents was to preserve and prolong childhood innocence, in part at least by the exercise of parental authority. More recently children have been allowed a degree of autonomy to exercise rights of their own. While children need care, nurturing and protection from danger, they also need to develop autonomy, good coping skills and competence. With a decreasing age of puberty and greater exposure to sex, violence and commerce at earlier ages through television, telephone and computer networks, children are acquiring a taste for what were formerly regarded as 'adult' experiences. Paradoxically, at the same time it is also apparent that children have more enforced dependency than ever before. They experience greater restriction on freedom of movement due to parental concerns about road accidents and dangers from strangers. They spend more years in school, experience exposure to the world of work at a later age, and are more dependent on parental financial support for longer than before. Thus transitions to adulthood have become prolonged at a time when children have demanded and received an earlier access to the adult world.[6] This has set up conflict in both adolescent and parental roles.

Thus, the task of bringing up a child is placing increased pressure on parents, who receive conflicting advice on the best childcare practices. Such pressure has also been augmented by new difficulties arising from the greater variety of family contexts and settings in which children are now raised. Children are brought up not only in the more traditional family structure involving two natural parents, but also in reconstituted families involving step-relationships, or by lone parents. Such family structures are relatively fluid: many parents realise there is a high likelihood that their children will experience more than one of these family types in their formative years. Thus parents have to be prepared to take responsibility not only for their own children, but also at times for their partners' children. Many parents may also have to cope with children reacting to damage suffered from a prior experience with another parent in a previous family setting. Thus the 'century of the child' is ending in ways unforeseen at its commencement, with significant implications for the role of parents.

CYCLES OF ABUSE

One of the effects that maltreatment in childhood can have on women is to impede their relationship with their own children. This was spontaneously commented on by the women we interviewed. For some women feelings of resentment about their childhood persisted and effectively paralysed their ability to relate to their own children. Although many women had sufficient insight to make the links between their past maltreatment and their current problems, tragically, some were unable to overcome them. One woman's story very clearly illustrates the effect that childhood maltreatment had on her relationship with her child. This particular woman felt that the repeated childhood rejections she experienced at the hands of her parents hampered her relationship with her own daughter. As a child she was farmed out to relatives and even the neighbours of relatives for years at a time, while her brothers and sisters remained living with their parents. Periodically she returned to her parents for short periods but was never shown any warmth or affection by either of them. She recounted a particularly hurtful incident which was typical of many she experienced: 'I was going on a school outing one day, and I kissed mum goodbye on the cheek – and the look of pure disgust on her face because I kissed her. Thank God I wasn't abused sexually, but it's what they did to me mentally that I find hard to understand.'

She reflected on the impact this had on her relationship with her own daughter: 'I find it hard to express affection, I can't sit and cuddle her and kiss her and do all those sort of things. I'm frightened that with my daughter now, she's at that age where she's going to say to me "Oh, leave me alone." I don't want to be rejected again, not by my kids. The way things have happened in my childhood doesn't help me in a relationship. My husband knows what I've been through. But I find it hard to really open up to him or to say to him "I *do* care about you", because it's just not me. I can't – I'm frightened all the time that I'm going be knocked back. It's happened to me too many times to let it happen now.'

For other women, the experience of hostile parenting made them more determined to ensure that, even if they could not correct the damage that had been done to themselves in childhood, they would at the very least not repeat the experience on the next generation. They had gone to admirable lengths to bring their own children up in a more positive way. One woman described her feelings about parenthood: 'I don't just want to bring my daughter up, to put clothes on her back and food in her mouth. I want to make sure that she knows that she is loved and wanted so she'll be less psychologically damaged than I was.'

Much is written currently about the repetition of abuse from one generation to the next.[7] However, there is a difference between the inability to show affection described in the example above and outright neglect or abuse. Some women who were neglected or abused as children may go on to repeat these experiences with their own children. However, this is not the only route by which cycles of abuse are perpetrated, nor the most likely route. Belief in this simple repetition as the basis of intergenerational transmission is also dangerously stigmatising for the abused mothers themselves. Such an explanation fails to take into account the complexity of the picture.

Although we have not reported on the intergenerational transmission of abuse in this book, the following facts derived from our research have some bearing on women's parenting. First, we know that sexual abuse of girls is almost exclusively from males and in most cases from an adult living outside the household. Therefore an abused parent, particularly a mother, is highly unlikely to be directly responsible for such abuse of her own children. Second, we know that the more severe physical abuse is most often from a male parent figure, and that both neglect and physical abuse occur most often in step-parent households. Therefore abuse occurring from one generation to the next is not necessarily through blood relatives. We also know that single-parent households, which are usually headed by the mother, have low rates of neglect or abuse during that arrangement. Finally, we have also learned that families in which neglect and abuse occur are those which suffer poverty, marital disharmony and parental psychiatric disorder. Therefore to point solely to a mother who was abused in childhood as the likely cause of a child's neglect or abuse is clearly misinformed.

However, since there is evidence for neglect and abuse crossing generations there must be some sense in which a mother can be a 'stress-carrier' for the conditions under which it can occur. One source is through her choice of partner. We know that women who suffered neglect or abuse in childhood are more likely to be in unsupportive partnerships or to have been separated from partners. As a result of their own childhood abuse, these women may be less discerning in adult relationships and quickly settle down with a partner who turns out to be less than ideal. This then increases risks for their children when marital breakdown results.

We have also shown that circumstances which give rise to depression in adult women are very similar to those which give rise to neglect and abuse of children. Both are highly adverse situations involving material hardship, unhappy marriages and partners' alcohol problems. Vulnerability to depression may thus be carried across generations not specifically through the parenting of a particular vulnerable individual such as the mother, but by a combination of poor choice of partner and greater proneness to adverse situations. Clearly the next step in researching these elements is to explore parenting, not only among vulnerable women but also their partners.

Research is currently under way in our team to examine such intergenerational links between the experience of childhood abuse and adult depression. To this end we are currently interviewing some of the mothers of the women who originally took part in our research. We aim to collect information about their approach to child-rearing, and to assess the pressures they experienced at the time of raising their children, including material hardship and unsupportive partners. We are assessing their own childhood experience as well, to see which, if any of these factors, has contributed to the neglect and abuse experienced by their daughters, the original research participants. We have also returned to re-interview some of the women themselves to ask about the way they and their partner have brought up their children, and assess the circumstances under which this occurred. To complete the picture, we are interviewing a group of their teenage children – young men as well as young women this time – to ask them about their experience of being raised by parents who were themselves abused as children. From this jigsaw puzzle of data it may be possible to predict vulnerable parenting style and link this with some of the other complex causes of child abuse.

SUMMARY AND IMPLICATIONS OF THE RESEARCH

We have surveyed in this book a range of childhood experiences which have had a dramatic effect on the lives of women. In the course of this research we have carefully defined and distinguished a number of types of childhood maltreatment and developed a method of assessing and grading them for severity. We have then been able to show that abusive experiences at the upper thresholds are significant in terms of being associated with depression in adult life.

The consequences of adverse early experience are far-reaching. While depression was our primary interest, we have also reported the effects neglect and abuse have on other aspects of psychological well-being including self-esteem and coping, and the ability to form supportive relationships across the life span. Childhood maltreatment has implications not only for the whole life course of the individual, but also across generations. Emotionally damaged children can enter adulthood ill-equipped to form close bonds, not only with other adults but also with their own children. Thus, the cycle of disadvantage may be continued, as parents unwittingly find themselves repeating the situations in which both depression and neglect of children are likely to flourish.

Undoubtedly, the experience of any type of abuse is detrimental to the psychological health of the individual in later life. In this respect we do not regard one type of abuse as necessarily more damaging than another. Other researchers and professionals often focus on the negative impact of a single type of experience, at times to the exclusion of all others. Thus at any given time one form of abuse appears more 'fashionable' or newsworthy than another. Yet in the course of writing this book we have seen media debate rise and fall over a host of issues: recovered memories of sexual abuse; neglected children left 'home alone'; legal rights to physically punish children; scandals concerning the multiple abuse of hundreds of children in institutional settings; calls for registration of convicted paedophiles; and limits on the availability of handguns following the massacre of school children at Dunblane. All of these causes and debates are equally important for the issue of child protection and since we know that many children are vulnerable to multiple forms of abuse from a number of perpetrators, all need to be tackled equally. While not wishing to undermine the seriousness of suffering a single type of abuse, the significance of experiencing a range of abuses needs to be stated. The women in our sample who experienced the combination of neglect, physical *and* sexual abuse had the worse outcomes in adulthood, although fortunately this was only a small minority of women.

Although our results show that maltreatment in childhood doubles the probability of becoming depressed in later life, this finding should not be interpreted fatalistically. As already discussed, around one in three with childhood adversity became depressed in the year of interview compared with one in ten of inner-city women in general. This has two implications. First, women *without* an adverse childhood can also become depressed, albeit less often. Second, the *majority* of women with adverse childhoods were not depressed and many spent considerable periods of their lives free of depression. Clearly much can happen in the intervening years between childhood and adulthood that will affect one's chances of becoming depressed, some of which may be a matter of simple good or bad luck, for example, in meeting a supportive or abusive partner.

Prevalence rates quoted throughout show that around a quarter or more of women in the community have experienced at least one type of neglect or abuse in childhood. Yet compared with some other estimates these maybe considered on the cautious side. This is because we have chosen a relatively high threshold for inclusion and only taken examples backed by evidence. Another reason is that the population which we have drawn upon to establish our prevalence figures is made up of women living in the community and, by definition, excludes certain groups, such as long-term psychiatric patients, prison populations or the homeless. Hence, those who are most damaged in terms of early experience may not be represented in our estimates.

NEW DIRECTIONS FOR RESEARCH

There are various topics this book has not covered simply because it was not within the remit of our research. When setting out to investigate topics as broad as childhood experience and adult mental health, it was necessary to be selective in what we studied. Some issues have been tackled in preference to others because of problems such as availability of subjects for study, complexity of research designs, or low prevalence of certain experience in the community at large. Some of the key issues which remain open to investigation are the role of gender, genetic contributions to depression, institutional abuse and the issue of other psychiatric disorders besides depression. Each of these will be discussed briefly in terms of future directions for related research into childhood neglect and abuse.

Gender

The present team has a history of focusing almost exclusively on the experience of women. The decision to explore the lives of women rather than men was guided by several factors. Not only is depression more common in women than in men, but it is also considerably easier to collect a representative sample of women to interview. Women are in general a less transient population than men, often being tied to a particular location by motherhood responsibilities and consequent use of health and educational services. Thus our methods of tracing women to interview through general practice surgeries has been an easier task than it would have been had we attempted to trace men of similar risk.

Documenting the experience of women as children and as mothers has been an important task to undertake, since during the course of this century women's roles have evolved with increasing complexity. Today's women are more likely to have sole responsibility for both the economic and emotional welfare of their children as evidenced by the increasing number of single mothers. At the same time, the high cost of living and need for personal development often require mothers to seek full-time employment. Thus for many women mothering responsibilities are greater than ever before, yet having sufficient time available to spend with their children is threatened.

However, it is equally clear that the research described here needs to be repeated with men. Initial work has already been carried out by other members of our team and shows that neglect and abuse are at similar levels among men and also influence psychiatric disorder. However, the outcome of such childhood maltreatment is as likely to include conduct disorder, anti-social personality disorder and substance abuse as depression. Further investigation is required to establish whether male psychiatric disorder arises from the same vulnerabilities that affect women. There is increasing evidence that for men disruption of roles involving work and non-domestic experiences have greater impact compared with the domestic crises that trigger women's depression.[8] There is also evidence that men view support differently: while at similar risk to women from a lack of support, men are more likely to receive support than to give it, creating inequalities for example in the marital relationship.[9] Understanding men's experiences is also crucial for a full understanding of women's experience since male behaviour has proved central to women's depressive experience. Lack of support from a partner (the majority of whom were male in our surveys), abuse from a partner, and partner's psychiatric or anti-social behaviour form part of the depressogenic experience for women. Further research is required to enhance understanding of the genesis of disorder in terms of partner choice and the resulting interaction between male and female vulnerability.

Genetics

Another topic which has not been discussed in the course of this book is the possible contribution of genetics to depression. There has been a revitalisation of interest in genetics following recent successes in the medical field. We have come a long way in beginning to understand the way in which social, psychological and developmental factors contribute to our understanding of childhood experience and adult depression. A final piece in the jigsaw could prove to be the interaction between genes for, say, temperament, and the environmental influences children encounter which produce vulnerability for later disorder. Recent interest in the possible links between genetic, social and developmental fields of investigation has led to a new research centre being established where collaborative work is being discussed.[10]

Since our own studies have focused on the measurement of environmental rather than genetic factors we can only hope to contribute to one particular part of the psychosocial picture. To test for a genetic influence in depression, genetic vulnerability factors would have to be assessed in conjunction with the psychological and environmental ones outlined. As with psychosocial vulnerability, such genetic tendencies will probably follow a similar model in requiring triggers from the environment through experiences such as maltreatment in childhood.

The psychosocial and genetic approaches are complementary rather than competing but require research designs with different characteristics. Our Sisters study, for example, with its emphasis on shared and non-shared environment in childhood, is similar to the type of design required for genetic research. However, a wider variety of sibling relationships needs to be involved in order to investigate both shared environment and shared genes. In particular, identical versus non-identical twins are required to judge heritability. The research methods discussed in this book would potentially be applicable to such designs.

In addition to genetic influences on disorder, there is also a role played by physiology. Neuroendocrinological differences have been observed between individuals who have suffered depression and those who remain depression free.[11] Thus, collaborative research is currently under way in our team to assess whether cortisol levels mirror patterns of psychosocial risk in adult women, and could add to the prediction of those who will become depressed.

Institutional abuse

The focus of this book has been primarily the treatment that children are exposed to while living with parents or replacement parents in the home. What has been omitted is the treatment of childhood in a variety of institutional settings such as care homes, hospitals, boarding schools, detention centres and reform schools. This is because of the relatively small numbers of such experiences in our series. The same forms of maltreatment are doubtless committed in such institutions, as evidenced by the host of abuse allegations uncovered in children and young people's care homes in recent years. At the time of writing, yet another scandal concerning the abuse of children in institutions in the North of England has been uncovered. This showed that scores of children were abused in the 1970s in homes targeted by paedophile 'carers'.

While there are no reliable estimates for the prevalence rates for abuse in these institutions, it seems that such abuse is not uncommon and an alarming aspect of institutional abuse is the greater numbers of children affected. Thus hundreds of children passing through an institution can be damaged by repeated abuse committed by a handful of abusers, with devastating long-term effects for the children. This is not to say that all care in institutions is detrimental to the child. Several of the women in our samples received good care in such settings. Indeed some described life in such homes as infinitely preferable to life in their parental home. Clearly general safeguards are needed for children to protect them from the adult abuse of power whether in family, school, youth clubs, church or institutional settings.

A range of psychiatric outcomes

For the sake of simplicity, the main outcome discussed throughout has been depression in the year of interview. In the course of interviews however, we collected a wealth of information regarding the duration and severity of episodes of depression occurring across the whole lifespan. Studies by our team have shown, for example, that women who suffer depression lasting continuously for a year or more are more likely to have experienced childhood neglect or abuse and early adult abuse.[12] These individuals are more handicapped by their symptoms than those with briefer episodes. General functioning required for day-to-day life is impeded, more symptoms are experienced and recovery is harder to effect.

In the course of interviews we also collected information about other behaviours and disorders such as conduct disorder, self-injury and suicide attempts, eating disorders, anxiety disorders, drug and alcohol abuse, all of which we are currently analysing in relation to childhood maltreatment. We are planning to add post-traumatic stress disorder in future research, which is particularly pertinent to the exploration of neglect and abuse in childhood. This disorder, identified with shell-shock among combat veterans and 'battered woman's syndrome' is a variant of anxiety particularly tied to life-threatening and abusive situations. It involves symptoms such as flashbacks or reliving of the trauma through nightmares.[13] These are symptoms which some women spontaneously recounted in the course of interviews.

CONCLUSION

Many politicians and journalists seek to label the family as the source and solution to a number of society's problems. They are quick to blame parents – single mothers, working mothers, absent fathers and so on. We have outlined in this book how a complex web of social and individual factors is responsible for childhood maltreatment and psychiatric disorders, not all of which can be placed on the shoulders of parents. While we acknowledge that poor parenting significantly influences a child's chances of being neglected or abused and thus depressed, we take the broader view that the whole context which gives rise to such abuse needs to be tackled. In this instance the context includes not only features of the individual parent, including the presence of mental illness as well as their own history of childhood abuse, but also features of the situation they find themselves in, including poverty, unemployment, poor housing and difficult marriages. It is clear that what also needs to be taken into consideration is the long-term view: by unravelling the childhood factors leading to later adult depression it may be possible to reduce the risk for the next generation, not only of abuse but also of depression. In this way we may begin to help future generations develop 'the habit of happiness' from their earliest years. As we approach the millennium we hope that lessons learned from this century of childcare may be carried over and superseded in the next.

NOTES

1   Cunningham, H. (1995) *Children and Childhood in Western Society since 1500*, London and New York: Longman.
2   Ennew, J. (1986) *The Sexual Exploitation of Children*, Cambridge: Polity.
3   Cunningham, op. cit. note 1.
4   Report of the National Commission of Inquiry into the Prevention of Child Abuse (1996) *Childhood Matters*, London: The Stationery Office.
5   Rosen, M. (1994) *The Penguin Book of Childhood*, London: Penguin.
6   Pilcher, J. (1995) *Age and Generation in Modern Britain*, Oxford: Oxford University Press.
7   Madge, N. (ed.) (1983) *Families at Risk*, London: Heinemann Educational.
8   Nazroo, J., Edwards, A. and Brown, G.W. (1997) 'Gender differences in the onset of depression following a shared life event: a study of couples', *Psychological Medicine 27*: 9–19.
9   Edwards, A., Nazroo, J. and Brown, G.W. (1997) 'Gender difference in marital support following a shared life event', *Social Science and Medicine* (in press).
10 The Social, Developmental and Genetic Research Centre, Camberwell, is directed by Michael Rutter and funded by the Medical Research Council.
11 Goldberg, D. and Huxley, P. (1992) *Common Mental Disorders: A Bio-social Model*, London, New York: Routledge.
12 Brown, G.W. and Moran, P. (1994) 'Clinical and psychosocial origins of chronic depressive episodes, I: a community survey', *British Journal of Psychiatry 165:* 447–456.
13 Herman, J. (1992) *Trauma and Recovery*, London: Pandora; USA: Basic Books.

Description of samples

The four studies referred to in this book were all of women living in the community in north London and selected through their registration with local general practices. All the studies were retrospective in the sense that childhood experiences were collected through their memories of early life. However, while two were solely retrospective and covered lifespan experience for women largely selected for adverse childhood experience (Loss of Mother and Sisters series) the other two had additional prospective components whereby women selected to a greater or lesser extent for vulnerability were followed up over a one- or two-year period to chart new onsets of disorder (Representative London Women and Adult Risk series). The four studies are described below in chronological order.

1 LOSS OF MOTHER STUDY (1977–80)

This study focused on women in the community who had experienced loss of or separation from a parent in childhood. The purpose of the study was to investigate a finding which had emerged from earlier research in Camberwell in the early 1970s conducted by George Brown and Tirril Harris, which showed that the loss of a mother in childhood acted as a vulnerability factor for depression in adult life. The women screened were aged 18–65 and registered with general practices in north-east London. All were sent a screening questionnaire to determine loss of either parent before the age of seventeen by death or separation for twelve months or more continuously. The response rate to nearly 3,000 questionnaires was 55 per cent. An investigation of non-responders from the first third of the series showing most were not at the addresses registered in the surgeries. If these are excluded the response rate was just under

70 per cent (this was to hold fairly constant for all subsequent screenings in the remaining studies). Of those replying to the questionnaire, 15 per cent indicated they had lost a parent before the age of seventeen. The refusal rate for being interviewed after returning a questionnaire was 10 per cent. In all, 225 women were selected and given lengthy interviews. Of these, 139 women experienced loss of a mother by death or separation and 41 experienced loss of a father alone, while a further 45 women had no parental loss.[1]

All women were given a lengthy face-to-face interview in their own home, in which they were asked about their childhood experience, early adult lives, current relationships and coping using an early version of the Self-Evaluation and Social Support instrument, and history of depression based on the Present State Examination (see Appendix II for description of interview measures). At this stage the 'Childhood Experience of Care and Abuse' (CECA) interview was in its early development and questioning revolved mainly around care and neglect. Abuse was added to the instrument at a later date. Therefore most of the interview and subsequent analyses concerned experiences surrounding the parental loss and the neglect which followed it. (In earlier publications this is termed 'lack of care' and as well as neglect involved lax supervision. The latter experience proved not to contribute additionally in later analyses.) The key finding to emerge was that 'lack of care' or neglect was more highly related to depression than the maternal loss. However, such lack of care was highly associated with maternal loss. Other findings showed that a number of experiences proved to be *unrelated* to adult depression, including discord in the home, the degree of practical change in childhood, and the mourning ritual and responses to maternal bereavement.[2]

In terms of adult risk factors mediating between childhood neglect and depression, the study found that premarital pregnancy, the presence of an unsupportive and unreliable partner, and poor coping in terms of helplessness were significant experiences.

2 REPRESENTATIVE LONDON WOMEN (1980–5)

A study was conducted among a largely consecutive series of working-class mothers aged 18–50 to examine adult vulnerability to depression. This utilised a prospective design to examine new onsets of disorder to ensure non-contamination of the vulnerability factors by depression. The study was conducted prospectively over two consecutive twelve-month follow-up periods. Women were selected for a somewhat raised risk of becoming depressed in terms of their demographic characteristics. Thus working-class women living in an inner-city area were chosen as depression is known to be higher in such groups. Single mothers were included regardless of their social class because of their similarly documented higher rates of depression. As in the earlier study, women were screened from the registers of general practitioners. Response rates to questionnaires were similar to those found in the Loss of Mother study (47 per cent). Again it was shown that non-responders were usually not living at the address listed in the doctors' records and that if excluded the effective response rate was around 70 per cent.[3]

Of the women who returned questionnaires around 20 per cent were demographically suitable. Again a relatively low rate of 7 per cent refused to be interviewed when contacted and nearly 400 women were interviewed in total. One year later 350 agreed to be seen for a second time. Of these nearly 50 were depressed at first interview and therefore the first twelve-month follow-up population referred to when discussing *new* onsets of disorder is 303 (chapters 9 and 10). Among these, 10.5 per cent (32) of women had onsets of depression during the follow-up year. It was thus possible to identify characteristics of vulnerability which existed prior to an onset of depression in the follow-up period.

At the first interview women were asked the 'Self-Evaluation and Social Support' interview schedule to assess a variety of factors hypothesised as increasing vulnerability for depression. Thus relationships with partner, children and other support figures were fully explored in addition to attitudes about the self including self-esteem. At both first and follow-up interviews the 'Present State Examination' was used to assess depressive symptomatology in the period between interviews. Finally an assessment of 'Life Events and Difficulties' was made covering the follow-up period, along with details of crisis support and coping with any events that had occurred.

The resulting model showed that the presence of low self-esteem, chronic subclinical conditions of depression or anxiety, interpersonal conflict with partner or child or lack of a close confidant (for those not living with a partner) increased risk of depression. (In order to simplify the analysis, chronic subclinical conditions and conflict with children have not been referred to in this book. However, similar results held when lack of support from partner or other close person and low self-esteem alone wére utilised.) These prior factors related to increased risk of depression only when a severe life event was encountered. Half the women had such vulnerability and half experienced a severe life event, but only a fifth experienced the combination of vulnerability *and* severe life event. The rate of depression among this relatively small group of 48 women was 45 per cent.

Childhood experience was collected using the full 'Childhood Experience of Care and Abuse' (CECA) instrument. This was used only at the time of *third* contact on 286 women, although summary assessments of loss of parent, antipathy and neglect had been collected on the full 400. Thus the smaller group is mainly quoted in this book. This group proved to be no different from the full series in terms of demographic characteristics or risk factors. This smaller group with full childhood histories has been utilised when referring to prevalence rates in earlier chapters. The prevalence of either neglect or abuse was 29 per cent and the experience of any one of the three (neglect, physical abuse or sexual abuse) doubled the rate of depression. Around a third with such childhood experience became depressed in the full three-year study period. Childhood neglect or abuse was found to be related to adult vulnerability and this explained its association with adult depression. In other words, its role in depression was solely mediated by ongoing low self-esteem and poor interpersonal relationships.

Early adult adversity was assessed in terms of experience of violence in cohabiting relationships or any sexual assault after age seventeen among the 286 women seen at third contact. Prevalences proved highly similar to the childhood experience: under a third experienced violence or sexual assault, though violence was more than twice as common as sexual assault. The experience of either doubled the likelihood of experiencing depression in the study period.

3 THE ADULT RISK SERIES (1990–5)

A partial replication of the Representative series was conducted, but this time only involving mothers with current vulnerability in order to assess if the one-in-three rates of onset of depression could be predicted from the previously identified vulnerability factors. Again this was a prospective study, this time following women over a fifteen-month period, during which there were follow-up contacts at around five and ten months. Screening for participants was again conducted through local general practice registers, where 3,000 questionnaires were sent out to women aged between eighteen and fifty eliciting a response rate almost identical to the earlier studies. From those who replied only working-class mothers or single mothers were selected, constituting half of the questionnaire replies. Of the remainder it was necessary to discard those already depressed at either major or minor level (a quarter of the remaining responses) and those with clearly low scores on a screening questionnaire assessing poor interpersonal relationships (a further quarter). A telephone screening was then conducted on the remaining responders. Of these 61 per cent were verified as being suitable for the project in terms of being free from depression and also having the adult vulnerability factors (of negative interaction with partner or child and lack of a close confidant).[4]

We interviewed 110 women initially, and 105 women agreed to complete all three interviews. Of these 37 per cent became depressed in the follow-up period, confirming the expected rate of onset. Over half of the women (60/105) had experienced childhood neglect or abuse, a significantly higher rate than the 29 per cent in the unselected Representative London Women series. Nearly three-quarters of the women (73/105) experienced a severe life event in the follow-up period, and among these women nearly half became depressed (35/73). Two factors proved to be associated with a lower risk of depression even among such vulnerable women. One was a rating of 'good ability to make and maintain relationships' at first interview and the second was good coping conferred by high mastery, optimism or downplaying at the time of a severe event. Both had the effect of halving risk.

4 SISTERS SERIES (1990–5)

This study was concurrent to the Adult Risk study and sought to explore further the role of *early* experience in relation to the sequence of adversity, vulnerability and depression occurring over the life course. It had the added aspect of including sister pairs in order to help determine the validity of the childhood accounts, and also to assess the degree to which sisters brought up in the same household had similar experiences.

Again women were selected through registration with general practices in north London, and of 4,000 questionnaires sent out, the usual response rate applied. The selection criteria for the first half of the sample involved having a sister no more than five years older or younger, who was brought up in the same household, was living in the UK and willing to be interviewed. Only 6 per cent of women proved suitable in terms of the selection criteria. The second half of the sample was selected by questionnaire screening mainly for the experience of parental neglect or antipathy in childhood before the age of seventeen, but including open-ended questions about other negative experience which elicited spontaneous reports of abuse. Again a suitable sister had to agree to be interviewed. The sample ultimately consisted of 40 pairs who were unselected and 60 pairs where the first in the pair reported childhood adversity. Of the initial questionnaire responders, 2 per cent refused to be interviewed and 13 per cent of co-sisters refused to be seen.[5]

The 40 consecutive pairs proved to be fairly representative of the north London population with rates of childhood neglect or abuse of 20 per cent (16/80) and adult depression in the year before interview 16 per cent (13/80) little different from the earlier Representative series. In some ways this group was more representative of the population at large since they were not selected for social class or motherhood status as in the Representative series. Three-quarters (62/80) were middle class, over half married (48/80) and half with children (43/80). Only 15 per cent (12/80) were single mothers when we interviewed them. Most were employed: 84 per cent (67/80).

The second group, consisting of women selected for reporting childhood adversity on the questionnaire, were little different in demographic terms from the unselected group: two-thirds were middle class (73/118), half (61/118) married, half (60/118) had children and 15 per cent (18/118) single mothers. Again most were employed: 75% (89/118). In many of the figures presented in earlier chapters the sisters have been combined into a single non-paired analysis. This was deemed legitimate since the two sister groups did not differ from each other in any demographic terms (social class, age, marital or motherhood status) nor in terms of risk status (low self-esteem, poor support or childhood adversity) or rates of depression. Significantly, despite having highly similar childhood experiences (a correlation of 0.60 for any severe neglect, physical or sexual abuse) there was no association between sisters for depression in the year of interview (correlation of 0.10). Therefore use of sisters could not have biased the relationship between childhood adversity and adult depression. The same results basically held if only one woman per family was utilised, but they have been combined here to give greater numbers and power of analysis.

The main aims of the study were first to confirm that parental neglect, physical and sexual abuse were related to adult depression. The second aim was to explore childhood in more detail, assessing role-reversal, psychological abuse, family context of abuse, childhood coping and response to adversity. Third, the study aimed to use the sister pairings to investigate the effects of shared and non-shared environment on outcome in sister pairs and to validate the accounts of childhood by asking each sister about the other and comparing accounts. Finally, we aimed to explore life-time consequences of such neglect or abuse in terms of the quality of close relationships, the extent of adult stressors, self-esteem, adult depression and other disorders.

It was confirmed that childhood adversity in terms of parental neglect, physical or sexual abuse doubled the risk of adult depression. This formed the simplest model: other related factors such as role-reversal, antipathy and psychological abuse did not assist prediction. Corroboration between sisters was in general very high and confirmed that the memories of adversity as measured by the CECA instrument appeared accurate. There was also a high degree of shared environment between sisters. This was particularly high for household abuse (neglect, physical and sexual) but low for sexual abuse from non-household members. It was also lower for antipathy from mother where favouritism or scapegoating of one daughter over the other was common.

Adult experiences shown to mediate between childhood neglect or abuse and adult depression in previous studies were confirmed with stressful teenage pregnancy, unsupportiveness of partner or lack of a confidant and low self-esteem all relating to both childhood experience and depression.

NOTES

1 Harris, T.O., Brown, G.W. and Bifulco, A. (1986) 'Loss of parent in childhood and adult psychiatric disorder: the role of lack of adequate parental care', *Psychological Medicine 16*: 641–659.
2 Bifulco, A., Harris, T.O. and Brown, G.W. (1992)'Mourning or inadequate care? Re-examining the relationship of maternal loss in childhood with adult depression and anxiety', *Development and Psychopathology 4*: 433–449.

3 Brown, G.W., Craig, T.K.J. and Harris, T.O. (1985) 'Depression: disease or distress? Some epidemiological considerations', *British Journal of Psychiatry 147*: 612–622.
4 Bifulco, A., Moran, P., Brown, G.W., Ball, C. and Campbell, C. (1998) 'Predicting depression in women: the role of past and present vulnerability', *Psychological Medicine* (in press).
5 Bifulco, A., Brown, G.W., Lillie, A. and Jarvis J. (1997) 'Memories of neglect and abuse: corroboration in a series of sisters', *Journal of Child Psychology and Psychiatry 38*: 365–374.

Instruments used

1 ASSESSMENT OF DEPRESSION: PRESENT STATE EXAMINATION (PSE)[1]

We defined depression in terms of recognised criteria established in a number of research studies, comparable to 'major depression' in psychiatric terminology. In practice this meant the presence of a cluster of symptoms which necessarily included depressed mood, defined as an uncontrollable, despairing, unhappy mood that couldn't be lifted by distractions or in company, often accompanied by crying and lasting most of the time. This, together with at least four other key symptoms constituted a 'clinical' case of depression. These included hopelessness where the future was seen pessimistically as entirely bleak, suicidal thoughts or plans, and poor concentration shown by inhibited ability to read a magazine or watch a television programme without thoughts drifting off. Other symptoms included brooding as evidenced by worrying to the extent that it interfered with normal activities, and 'retardation' which involved a slowing down of movement, and perception of the rest of the world as moving too fast. Negative feelings about the self (for example feeling inferior or worthless) and the outside world (for example losing interest in enjoyable activities, appearance and home-making) were also present. Normal physical functions such as appetite and sleep were typically impaired, resulting in loss of weight, and inability to get off to sleep or remain asleep.

Five such symptoms, including depression, had to be present for at least half of any one month and for a minimum of four weeks in order to count as a 'case'-level depression. Depression at this level involved symptoms considered sufficiently severe and disabling to merit treatment by a psychiatrist. Only a minority who experienced such severe depression sought treatment (under a third), mostly by general practitioners but a small proportion from psychotherapists or psychiatrists. The majority of episodes of depression lasted three months or more, but as many as 45 per cent went on for over a year. In the Adult Risk series we also assessed depression by means of the American *DSM-IIIR* classification and found almost total overlap in the classification of cases.

2 CHILDHOOD EXPERIENCE OF CARE AND ABUSE (CECA)[2]

The CECA instrument has been described at length in the chapters in this book. To summarise: it is a detailed semi-structured interview about negative childhood experiences, requiring judgements to be made by the investigator about the information collected on the basis of a series of rules and precedent rating examples. The interview takes on average one hour to administer, although this of course varies according to the number of different parent figures in childhood and the number of abuses, with interview duration ranging from half an hour to over two hours. Training courses lasting four days are held twice a year in order to teach the administration and rating of the CECA. Each trainee is given an extensive manual with examples of threshold ratings and rules for inclusion.

Initial questions concern loss or separation from parent up to the age of seventeen. In this way the number of different family arrangements within which an individual was brought up is determined. The questions concerning care, antipathy of parents, discord and violence between parents are repeated for each of these family arrangements. All physical abuse from household members is covered, as well as all sexual abuse regardless of household membership. The Sisters series used a longer version of the CECA in order to explore additional experiences such as role-reversal and psychological abuse, together with family context involving financial hardship, parent's psychiatric disorder, etc.

What makes the instrument different from other measures of childhood is the breadth of coverage and the use of contextual judgements for assessing severity. Thus ratings of severity of sexual abuse are not based purely on the degree of sexual contact as in some other instruments, but also on a range of other contextual information such as relationship to the perpetrator, frequency of abuse, early age of abuse, imposed secretiveness and so on. This method has proved successful in succinctly capturing the full contextual severity of the experience. The reliability of the instrument is high, with correlations between independent raters on 20 interviews all above 0.78.

3 SELF-EVALUATION AND SOCIAL SUPPORT (SESS)[3]

In the SESS interview various assessments were made of the quality of close relationships and support, with particular focus on the partner and confiding relationships. Key scales covered confiding, emotional support and negative interaction. Lack of support as defined in the 'Negative Elements in Close Relationships' (NECR) index involved the absence of any close confidant for a single woman and high negative interaction for those living with a partner. Another aspect included in the index but not highlighted in this book was that of negative interaction with children in the home. Negative interaction involved discord, criticism, tension and, at worst, violence.

Self-evaluation was an index based on three scales: negative evaluation of personal attributes (such as attractiveness or intelligence), negative evaluation of competence in roles (for example as a mother or friend) or self-rejection (a more global assessment of self-dislike). These three scales were highly correlated but a high rating on any one would count as 'negative evaluation of self' (NES). Inter-rater reliability on both support and self scales was high with correlations of over 0.83.

4 EARLY ADULT ABUSE[4, 5]

There were two assessments of adult abuse which mirrored aspects of the CECA. The first involved violence from partner and was assessed, as in childhood, by the presence of beatings, hitting with implements or fists or threats to kill with the most common attacks involving punches, kicks and being beaten up. A quarter of women in the Representative London series reported having experienced violence from their partner at some point in their adult lives. Nearly all reported injuries including black eyes, bruising and at times broken noses. For two-thirds of the women the violence was repeated and regular.

The second type of adult abuse assessed was that of sexual assault. These were defined in terms of actual or attempted rape and most were accompanied by threats, coercion or force. As with childhood abuse these were less common than the experience of violence, with 8 per cent reporting at least one sexual assault in adulthood. In practice the largest proportion of assaults were from partners or boyfriends (50 per cent) with a quarter from other known men and a quarter from strangers.

5 LIFE EVENTS AND DIFFICULTIES (LEDs)[6, 7]

In the model of depression described here, the stressors required to act as provoking agents consisted of severe life events or major difficulties. Severe life events or crises are those judged by the interviewer to carry a 'marked' or 'moderate' degree of threat or unpleasantness, lasting at least two weeks from the beginning of the event. Such events include deaths of close others, partner's infidelity, children's delinquency, unplanned pregnancy or material crises such as redundancy or eviction. The type of events most likely to provoke a depression proved to be those involving close relationships. Characteristics of such severe events most related to onset are those likely to produce shame, such as humiliations, personal failures and stigmatising events.

Major difficulties are chronic stressors in similar categories which have lasted continuously for two years or more. Although these are less potent as provoking agents, a severe event arising out of such a difficulty greatly increases risk of onset and an 'entrapping' event is one of these. The LEDs has now been used extensively over the last twenty years by a number of teams studying both psychiatric and physical illness. Its inter-rater reliability is high with correlations of around 0.90 for assessing severity of life events.

NOTES

1 Wing, J.K., Cooper, J.E. and Sartorius, N. (1974) *The Measurement and Classification of Psychiatric Symptoms*, Cambridge: Cambridge University Press.
2 Bifulco, A., Brown, G.W. and Harris, T.O. (1994) 'Childhood Experience of Care and Abuse (CECA): a retrospective interview measure', *Child Psychology and Psychiatry 35*: 1419–1435.
3 Brown, G.W., Bifulco, A., Veiel, H. and Andrews, B. (1990) 'Self-esteem and depression, II: social correlates of self-esteem', *Social Psychiatry and Psychiatric Epidemiology 25*: 225–234.
4 Andrews, A. and Brown, G.W. (1988) 'Marital violence in the commu-

nity: a biographical approach', *British Journal of Psychiatry 153*: 305–312.

5 Brown, G.W., Harris, T.O. and Eales, M. (1993) 'Aetiology of anxiety and depressive disorders in an inner-city population, 2: comorbidity and adversity', *Psychological Medicine 23*: 155–165.

6 Brown, G.W. and Harris, T. (1978) *Social Origins of Depression*, London: Tavistock.

7 Brown, G.W., Harris, T. and Hepworth, C. (1995) 'Loss, humiliation and entrapment among women developing depression: a patient and non-patient comparison', *Psychological Medicine 25*: 7–21.

Index